Towards a Classless Societ

In recent years, the Right has made all the running in the debate over class, with its rhetoric of a classless society coupled with the notion of an underclass. It was not always so. 'Class' has been a long-standing tool of analysis for social commentators and historians of all shades of opinion, as well as an inspiration for fundamental social change.

By covering young people and their poverty; health, education and training; homelessness; youth crime and young single mothers, *Towards a Classless Society?* underlines the role played by the labour market in influencing an individual's life chances, and the way in which labour market position is closely linked to class position. While the interplay of class and labour market heavily influences young people's life chances, government policies operate on the assumption that young people's culture determines how successfully they will step up the class ladder. Governments operate within the constraints of a false analysis of the root causes of class inequalities, as well as a globalised economy, and long-term socio-economic trends. Social workers, the professionals who work most closely with the poorest and most vulnerable members of society, have found it suprisingly difficult to sustain any challenge to individualistic and cultural explanations for class inequalities.

Towards a Classless Society? provides an alternative to the right-wing paradigm that has hijacked discussions of class. By focusing on the specific ways in which class inequalities manifest themselves in 1990s Britain, it exposes the hollowness of politicians' rhetoric about the classless society.

Helen Jones lectures in Social Policy at Goldsmiths College, University of London.

The State of Welfare
Edited by Mary Langan

Nearly half a century after its post-war consolidation, the British welfare state is once again at the centre of political controversy. After a decade in which the role of the state in the provision of welfare was steadily reduced in favour of the private, voluntary and informal sectors, with relatively little public debate or resistance, the further extension of the new mixed economy of welfare in the spheres of health and education became a major political issue in the early 1990s. At the same time the impact of deepening recession has begun to expose some of the deficiencies of market forces in areas such as housing and income maintenance, where their role had expanded dramatically during the 1980s. The State of Welfare provides a forum for continuing the debate about the services we need in the 1990s.

Titles of related interest also in The State of Welfare Series:

The Dynamics of British Health Policy
Stephen Harrison, David Hunter and Christopher Pollitt

Radical Social Work Today
Edited by Mary Langan and Phil Lee

Taking Child Abuse Seriously
The Violence Against Children Study Group

Ideologies of Welfare: From Dreams to Disillusion
John Clarke, Allan Cochrane and Carol Smart

Women, Oppression and Social Work
Edited by Mary Langan and Lesley Day

Managing Poverty: The Limits of Social Assistance
Carol Walker

The Eclipse of Council Housing
Ian Cole and Robert Furbey

Towards a Post-Fordist Welfare State?
Roger Burrows and Brian Loader

Working with Men: Feminism and Social Work
Edited by Kate Cavanagh and Viviene E. Cree

Social Theory, Social Change and Social Work
Edited by Nigel Parton

Working for Equality in Health
Edited by Paul Bywaters and Eileen McLeod

Social Work and Child Abuse
Dave Merrick

Social Action with Children and Families
Edited by Crescy Cannan and Chris Warren

Child Protection and Family Support
Edited by Nigel Parton

Towards a Classless Society?

Edited by Helen Jones

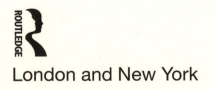

London and New York

First published 1997
by Routledge
11 New Fetter Lane, London EC4P 4EE

Simultaneously published in the USA and Canada
by Routledge
29 West 35th Street, New York, NY 10001

Typeset in Times by Routledge
Printed and bound in Great Britain by Redwood Books,
Trowbridge, Wiltshire

British Library Cataloguing in Publication Data
A catalogue record for this book is available from the British Library

Library of Congress Cataloguing in Publication Data
Towards a classless society? / edited by Helen Jones.
p. cm (The state of welfare)
Includes bibliographical references and index.
1. Social classes–Great Britain 2. Great Briain–Social policy. 3. Great
Britain–Economic policy. I. Jones, Helen, 1954–. II. Series.
HN400. S6T69 1997
305.5' 0941–dc21   97–9747
                                                              CIP

ISBN 0–415–15330–1 (hbk)
ISBN 0–415–15331–X (pbk)

Contents

Illustrations

Contributors

Fiona Devine is a Senior Lecturer in Sociology at the University of Manchester. She has published widely in the field of class analysis, including *Affluent Workers Revisited* (Edinburgh University Press, 1992) and *Social Class in America and Britain* (Edinburgh University Press, 1997). She is currently Chair of the Editorial Board of *Sociology* and an Associate Editor of *Gender, Work and Organisation.*

Andy Furlong is a Senior Lecturer in Sociology and Director of the Youth, Education and Employment Research Unit at the University of Glasgow. He is author of *Growing Up in a Classless Society?* (Edinburgh University Press, 1992), *Schooling for Jobs* (Avebury, 1993) *Young People and Social Change* with Fred Cartmel (Open University Press, 1997) and many articles on young people.

Susan Hutson is a Senior Lecturer at the University of Glamorgan. She has published widely in the field of homelessness, including *Youth Homelessness* with Mark Liddiard (Macmillan, 1994) and with Richard Jenkins *Taking the Strain* (Open University Press, 1989).

Chris Jones is Professor of Social Policy and Social Work at the University of Liverpool. Recent publications include 'Anti-intellectualism and the peculiarities of British social work education', in Nigel Parton (ed.) *Social Theory, Social Change and Social Work* (Routledge, 1996), and 'Dangerous times for British social work education', in Peter Ford and Patrick Hayes (eds) *Educating for Social Work* (Avebury, 1996).

Helen Jones lectures in Social Policy at Goldsmiths College, University of London. Her publications include *Health and Society in Twentieth-Century Britain* (Longman, 1994), *Social Policy and the*

City edited with John Lansley (Avebury, 1995) and *The Politics of the Family* edited with Jane Millar (Avebury, 1996).

Mark Liddiard lectures in social policy at the University of Kent. He is the co-author with Susan Hutson of *Youth Homelessness* (Macmillan, 1994) and has published widely in the field of homelessness. Currently he is working in the field of museums.

Tony Novak is a Lecturer in Social Policy at the University of Liverpool. He has researched and written a number of books and articles about various aspects of poverty, including its history and politics and the response of the state in Britain to the problems and challenges it provokes.

Robert Page lectures in Social Policy and Administration at the University of Nottingham. He is the author of *Stigma* (Routledge & Kegan Paul, 1984) and *Altruism and the British Welfare State* (Avebury, 1996); he has co-edited a number of books including *The Costs of Welfare* with Nicholas Deakin (Avebury, 1993) and *Modern Thinkers on Welfare* with Vic George (Prentice-Hall, 1995).

John Pitts has been a youth worker, an Intermediate Treatment Co-ordinator, and a group worker in a psychiatric Borstal. He has written extensively on youth crime and justice and is currently Professor of Socio-Legal Studies at the University of Luton.

Kenneth Roberts is Professor of Sociology at the University of Liverpool. Among his many publications he is the author or co-author of *Black Youth in Liverpool* (Giordano Bruno, 1991), *Careers and Identities* (Open University Press, 1992), *Youth and Employment in Modern Britain* (Oxford University Press, 1995), and *Poland's First Post-Communist Generation* (Avebury, 1995).

Series editor's preface

In the 1990s the perception of a crisis of welfare systems has become universal across the Western world. The coincidence of global economic slump and the ending of the Cold War has intensified pressures to reduce welfare spending at the same time that Western governments, traditional social institutions and political parties all face unprecedented problems of legitimacy. Given the importance of welfare policies in securing popular consent for existing regimes and in maintaining social stability, welfare budgets have in general proved remarkably resilient even in face of governments proclaiming the principles of austerity and self-reliance.

Yet the crisis of welfare has led to measures of reform and retrenchment which have provoked often bitter controversy in virtually every sphere, from hospitals and schools to social security benefits and personal social services. What is striking is the crumbling of the old structures and policies before any clear alternative has emerged. The general impression is one of exhaustion and confusion. There is a widespread sense that everything has been tried and has failed and that nobody is very clear about how to advance into an increasingly bleak future.

On both sides of the Atlantic, the agenda of free market anti-statism has provided the cutting edge for measures of privatisation. The result has been a substantial shift in the 'mixed economy' of welfare towards a more market-oriented approach. But it has not taken long for the defects of the market as a mechanism for social regulation to become apparent. Yet now that the inadequacy of the market in providing equitable or even efficient welfare services is exposed, where else is there to turn?

The *State of Welfare* series aims to provide a critical assessment of the policy implications of some of the wide social and economic

changes of the 1990s. Globalisation, the emergence of post-industrial society, the transformation of work, demographic shifts and
changes in gender roles and family structures all have major consequences for the patterns of welfare provision established half a
century ago.

The demands of women and minority ethnic groups, as well as
the voices of younger, older and disabled people and the influence
of social movements concerned with issues of sexuality, gender and
the environment must all be taken into account in the construction
of a social policy for the new millennium.

Mary Langan

Chapter 1

Introduction

Helen Jones

POPULAR PERCEPTIONS AND THE POLITICIANS

In 1996, when John Prescott, the Deputy Leader of the Labour Party, announced on the radio, 'I'm pretty middle-class', not all, including his father, agreed with him, and his throwaway remark fuelled a debate in the media over what it meant to be middle-class or working-class (see, for instance, the *Daily Telegraph*, 13 April 1996). Ideas of what determines a person's class position varied: was it 'breeding' or 'manners, courtesy and behaviour', as two callers to a Radio 4 phone-in programme, *Call Nick Ross*, suggested? While there are popular disagreements over definitions and classifications, it is still widely accepted that class exists in Britain; indeed, according to Gallup Poll surveys, an increasing percentage of the population think that there is a class struggle in progress (1961 56 per cent; 1981 66 per cent; 1991 79 per cent; autumn 1995 81 per cent).

Yet, from the time of his successful bid for the leadership of the Conservative Party in 1990, John Major portrayed himself as the classless Prime Minister, with a mission to create a classless society. He presented himself as the role model *par excellence* for a classless society as he personalised the political by trying to make political capital out of his humble origins: for instance in a party political television broadcast during the 1992 General Election campaign, which showed him driving past his childhood haunts in Brixton. He has been portrayed as a man who pulled himself up by his boot-straps, and this fits well with his vision of a classless society, for effort and reward play an important part in it. One of his biographers claimed that it was Major's own experience that prompted his desire for everyone to have the chance to rise from any background: what he achieved he wants to make possible for others (Ellis 1991).

His call is therefore for class mobility, not classlessness. The way in which John Major equates 'classlessness' with opportunity within a class-structured society was underlined at the 1996 Conservative Party Conference where he spoke, under the slogan 'Opportunity for All', of creating an 'opportunity-owning democracy' in which all people would have the 'opportunity and choice, to open up an avenue of hope in their lives'.

Major's vision of a classless society is not one in which structural class inequalities are removed, or resources distributed more equally. It was not the prospect of a radically different future that he held out, and indeed he went to great pains to emphasise the continuity of his vision with traditional conservatism, looking back to Disraeli rather than his immediate predecessor (Major 1993). (He had, of course, to establish himself quickly as his own man, with his own brand of Conservatism, if he was to avoid disappearing into the shadow of Mrs Thatcher.) Indeed, at first glance prioritising the goal of a 'classless' society would seem to represent a drastic departure from Mrs Thatcher's rhetoric; she did not believe in society, let alone a classless one.

Yet the shift was not so stark, for, along with his talk of a classless society, much of what John Major said was very much in keeping with Mrs Thatcher's Britain. He spoke of continuing to make changes in order to transform society into a classless one within a decade. Both he and Mrs Thatcher repeatedly referred to the importance of creating and sustaining an enterprise culture, one in which business acumen and hard work were rewarded. In the 1990s the priority that Mrs Thatcher had accorded to private business, to selling off state-owned concerns and injecting business methods into those areas that remained under the state, to a mixed economy of welfare, to reducing the powers of local authorities and trade unions, and to reducing the poor's alleged culture of dependency on the state remained unchanged. These were also the themes of John Major's colleagues, none of whom appeared interested in a classless society. Peter Lilley, for instance, chided the Church of England for speaking out on poverty, a subject which he considers to be no business of the Church. Nor does he accept that poverty is a problem in Britain; he sees it primarily as a problem of water and food supply in the Third World, and for this reason he saw no role for the British Government in the 1996 International Year for the Eradication of Poverty (*Guardian*, 17 April 1996, 14 June 1996).

Major has spoken of everyone having a stake in the future, of effort being rewarded and of people having more choice in the way they spend their money. His classless society is one in which people have the opportunity to spend more in a consumer society. (Since the power to choose to spend money requires having enough of it to participate in buying the same range of goods as the bulk of the population, it is illogical to suppose that one can create a classless society simply by creating more wealth, without redistributing it.)

Major sees young people playing a central role in creating a classless society. He has spoken of every youngster aiming high, and of making this possible by raising the esteem in which vocational qualifications are held; by removing prejudice and the hidden barriers to success; and by having successful women or people from ethnic minorities as role models.

Labour politicians took up the term 'classless society' as a stick with which to beat the Conservatives. 'Why has the man who promised a classless society set his face against plans that will make a reality of that classless society?' asked Tony Blair (*Independent*, 19 January 1996). Yet, Blair's rhetoric of creating a stakeholder society appears on the surface to be very similar to John Major's idea of a classless society with opportunity for all. Blair has spoken about the need for all to have a stake in society, of breaking down the barriers which hold people back, of building a meritocracy, and of creating the opportunities for wealth and power to be shared more widely. At the 1995 Labour Party conference he claimed that Britain was divided by an unfair class system, tattered social fabric and dogmatic politics. He spoke of unity, solidarity, and partnership. He emphasised the importance of education and of wanting to make Britain young again. His rhetoric has been concerned with giving more people the opportunity to share in wealth and power, creating economic and social stability and social cohesion which require that all citizens have a stake in society: his famous 'stakeholder society'. He has argued that a meaningful stake in society comes through the ability to earn a living and support a family. So there should be education, employment and community initiatives to slash youth unemployment; for single parents there should be a job, education and training programme. He has spoken of 'decent' nursery education and child-care provision, smaller infant class sizes, broader 'A' levels and upgraded vocational qualifications (*Renewal*, October 1995; *Guardian*, 29 January 1996).

Labour Party leaders, using similar terminology to the Conservatives, have accepted much of the Right's analysis of the causes of Britain's ills. There is a distinct possibility that the current vogue among politicians for a moral crusade against Sodom and Gomorrah will divert attention from the socio-economic structural inequalities that have contributed so much to Britain's social problems. On 15 October 1996, on the Radio 4 *Today* programme, Jack Straw, the then shadow spokesman on Home Affairs, would not admit that redistribution of wealth was part of the solution to the problem of pockets of high youth crime, but chose instead to reiterate Tony Blair's views, expressed the previous day in a speech in South Africa in which he called for the re-establishment of 'family values'.

In recent years, the Right has made all the running in the debate over class, with its rhetoric of a classless society coupled with the notion of an underclass – terminology now bandied about by politicians on all sides. It was not always so. 'Class' has been a long-standing tool of analysis for social commentators and historians of all shades of opinion, as well as an inspiration for fundamental social change.

THE ACADEMIC DEBATE

Current social classifications and ways of analysing the stratification of society all build on, refine or refute Marx's and Weber's nineteenth-century analyses. For Marx, class position is determined by an individual's or group's relationship to the means of production, and class relations always involve exploitation and domination. The image is that of a see-saw: as one class goes up the other must inevitably go down. For Weber, the relationship between classes more closely resembles a sliding scale. He argued that class position was determined by a person's place in the market, which is influenced by education and skills, rather than by their relationship to the system of production. Weber also claimed that a person's class position was influenced not only by the economic system but also by status and group power within a hierarchical society. Whereas Marx saw the working class and middle class locked in conflict, Weber saw classes as separate, hierarchical structures, but not necessarily in conflict.

As Rosemary Crompton and others have pointed out, post-war writers, such as Dahrendorf and Lockwood, have focused on the occupational structure or, like Bourdieu, have argued that consumption and lifestyles are the key determinants of class. Various attempts have also been made to integrate gender and ethnicity into class schema (Miliband 1989). While there are those who argue that the working class has joined the middle class and become indistin-guishable from it (the embourgeoisement thesis), or that a section of the working class has dropped out of the class system altogether and become a new underclass, class continues to provide the key tool for analysing stratification in today's society. Neither Marx's nor Weber's image of a classless society has been achieved. For Marx, this would occur when the working class had overthrown the capitalist class and private property had been abolished; for Weber, it would occur when privilege, and differentiation based upon it, had given way to equality of opportunity (for general discussions of class see Crompton 1993; Edgell 1993; Kelsall, Kelsall and Chisholm 1984).

TOWARDS A CLASSLESS SOCIETY?

Popular and academic views on the continuing relevance of class are in close accord, as the contributors to this volume make clear. The following chapters provide an alternative to the right-wing paradigm that has hijacked discussions of class, and, by focusing on the specific ways in which class inequalities manifest themselves in 1990s Britain, they expose the hollowness of politicians' rhetoric about the classless society.

The chapters in this volume underline the key role played by the labour market in influencing an individual's life chances, and the way in which labour-market position is closely linked to class posi-tion. While the interplay of class and labour market heavily influences young people's life chances, Government policies operate on the assumption that young people's culture, their behaviour and mores, determines how successfully they will step up the class ladder. Governments operate within the constraints of a false analysis of the root causes of class inequalities, as well as a glob-alised economy, and long-term socio-economic trends. If the analysis is fundamentally flawed, it is hardly surprising that Government solutions, at best, are irrelevant and, at worst, reinforce young people's class-related life chances and marginalise broad swathes of Britain's youth. Politicians have adopted a somewhat simplistic definition of a 'classless society', but – even judged on this narrow definition – there is no evidence that the next generation will find itself in a classless Britain. The links between poverty and class-related inequalities are underlined by various contributors. The pervasiveness of class inequalities are such that one in three children in Britain is growing up in poverty. Such children therefore have the double burden of living with the material and cultural deprivation of poverty, and also of struggling within a class society.

In Chapter 2 Tony Novak provides an overview of growing inequalities and the extent of poverty among children and young people, and addresses a number of the themes taken up in subsequent chapters. He points to the labelling of young people who are Black, single parents or unemployed (and, of course, it is possible to fall into all three categories at once) as an underclass living in a counter-cultural world into which they have supposedly voluntarily stepped, whereas, in fact, their mores are much the same as those of mainstream society. Novak argues that this false representation is an attempt to square the circle of growing class-related inequalities and extensive poverty in a society that is supposedly becoming classless.

In Chapter 3 Helen Jones continues the theme of class inequalities and poverty, reviewing the wealth of evidence that exists of the continuing importance of class position in determining a child's or young person's health and well-being, and of the negative effects of poverty on standards of health and well-being.

In Chapter 4 Andy Furlong demonstrates that, as with health, so with educational attainment, class inequalities are not diminishing. He argues that middle-class cultural capital is still important. Furlong, however, points to the weakening influence of class for the educational attainment of girls and young women, for whom participation in the labour market has grown in significance, and so, consequently, has the need for appropriate qualifications to enable them to compete effectively in it. The significance of the labour market for all young people, and the fear of unemployment, has meant an increasingly individualised (rather than a group) response to the education system, and more subtle challenges to that system.

Knuckling-down and working within the system does not, however, bring automatic success; in Chapter 5 Ken Roberts details the ways in which youth training schemes have been weakened by influences well beyond the remit of the schemes themselves and, in particular, by the absence of a policy of full employment.

Weaknesses in the labour market as well as in the housing market have hit young people disproportionately hard, according to Susan Hutson and Mark Liddiard in Chapter 6. Over many years a range of Government policies has reinforced the marginalised position of young people in society, and those already in a weak position have had their problems compounded.

In Chapter 7 John Pitts argues that socio-economic and policy changes have all conspired to throw the poor young (often young mothers) together on the most deprived council estates, where many young people have a criminal lifestyle that they do not grow out of. He contrasts British criminal and penal policy responses with French initiatives, which have tried to create a new social solidarity and new routes into citizenship.

Robert Page, in Chapter 8, focuses on young single mothers, who have suffered from a revival in centuries-old prejudices and remain marginalised as citizens. Government policies aim to change young girls' behaviour in order to discourage young single motherhood, but this has had the effect of further stigmatising and marginalising them.

The problem of focusing on individual behaviour, rather than the structural causes of class inequalities and poverty, is also Chris Jones's theme in Chapter 9. He argues that social workers, the professionals almost exclusively concerned with poor people, have failed to publicise the consequences of an increasingly unequal society. They have played down the significance of the material context of poverty while emphasising individual and family behaviours. When social workers did point to the systemic failures of society, they suffered an onslaught from the Conservative Government and the media, and public vilification and changes in social work training meant that they were in no position to present a forceful and convincing critique of poverty and inequality.

In Chapter 10 Fiona Devine looks at the future prospects for a classless society. Given the past record of governments she is not optimistic. Like previous contributors, she emphasises the importance of the labour market for reducing class inequalities. She argues that in the past life chances have only been made more equal when there has been economic growth, thus avoiding the need for redistribution of wealth and income in order to create greater opportunity. In reviewing past governments' performances, and the current claims of all three political parties, she points to politicians' limited vision of a classless society: for politicians, equal opportunities are about the way in which unequal rewards are distributed, and this only ensures that class inequalities continue.

Creating a classless society needs a well-thought-out strategy, with specific policies for reducing poverty and extensive class-related inequalities. While Britain can learn from the experiences and responses of other European countries, policies need to be generated from within Britain, for, although Eurosceptics look with horror, and Euro-enthusiasts with hope, to the prospect of a more integrated Europe, its implications for poverty and inequality in Britain are strictly circumscribed.

The EU and young people

EU social policies are primarily aimed at those in employment. The Social Affairs Directive sees the promotion of employment in the EU as a means of including marginalised groups (the rhetoric is not unlike that of politicians of all colours in Britain). Calls are made for those most in need to receive priority, the opposite of the 'trickle-down effect'. In reality, EU social policies are very narrowly conceived. Even if Britain had signed up to the Social Chapter, it would have had little effect beyond the workplace, because it focuses on rights at work; it is therefore of little relevance to tackling either the underlying causes of poverty or the problem of those who are not part of the formal labour force. Many children and young people do, of course, undertake paid work, and this is one area where an EU directive on the rights and protection of children and adolescents could be directly relevant. Although the Directive's main aim is to prevent the employment of children, there are numerous exceptions, however, and the unreality of banning child employment is recognised in its various stipulations about their hours of work, night work, rest periods, leave and rest breaks. It fails to address the underlying reasons why children have to work when this is widely regarded as undesirable (European Commission 1994: 302–3).

The limitations of EU social policy for reducing poverty and class inequalities in Britain are clear, while any attempts to bring public spending down to levels suitable for joining the single currency would be likely to aggravate inequalities and reduce the amount of state welfare. Yet one of the arguments in favour of joining the single currency is that it would act as a buffer for Britain against international competition: a matter of increasing concern in the globalised economy. As multinational companies look away from Europe for cheaper sources of labour, Britain must respond by offering high-quality products, not by reducing wages to third-world levels in order to produce shoddy, third-rate goods. Peter Townsend (1992: 1) has called for multinational collaboration and action as a future basis for an effective approach to social policies, but widespread action of this nature lies far in the future. Britain has to look to social policies which are within its control if it is to protect the most vulnerable and make any progress towards a classless society. What policies and projects are on offer?

Labour Party plans

John Smith, when leader of the Labour Party, pledged that his party would establish a Children's Commissioner, but Tony Blair has made no such commitment. It seems that Labour has dropped a commitment to restore the link between benefit levels and earnings, and it has announced that there will be no increase in welfare spending (*Guardian*, 4 June 1996; *Observer*, 11 August 1996). It seems, too, that it intends to exclude those under 18 from any statutory minimum wage, because of the 30 per cent rise in unemployment in this age group. This exclusion would be offered to employers as a trade-off for being required to allow 16- and 17-year-olds one day a week off for training.

The Labour Party has, however, offered a number of alternative plans which will directly affect children and young people. First, it has a plan, called Target 2000, which envisages ending Youth Training and replacing it with a new Youth Training guarantee. The money will come from a one-off tax on public utilities and from savings from abolishing YT. Second, as part of the public spending review of post-16 education financing undertaken by Gordon Brown, David Blunkett and Chris Smith, the idea is being floated of abolishing child benefit for 16- to 18-year-olds (*Guardian*, 22 April 1996). Third, after leaving school every teenager should have an individual learning account, and everyone will be entitled to a certain amount of financial support from the state at some point in their careers. This is seen as part of a strategy for lifelong opportunities for all and a commitment to equal opportunities (*Guardian*, 19 April 1996). Fourth, it has been suggested that the policy of some Local Education Authorities (LEAs) of permitting education and training outside school for disaffected young people who have not reached the school leaving age should be extended to all LEAs. Such young people should follow part of their studies at a Further Education college working closely with local businesspeople. Courses should be more relevant, and all students should receive extensive work experience. One problem with this scheme is that it may come to be regarded as a sink for those children who do not do well at school, and colleges may resent having the most alienated children dumped on them (*Guardian*, 19 March 1996). Whether in fact Blair's rhetoric does signify a move towards a classless society can only be judged by Labour policies in power.

PROPOSALS

The contributors to this volume have identified key areas which should be the basis of social policies for any government that is seriously committed to moving towards a classless society. Susan Hutson and Mark Liddiard argue that marginalised young people, in particular the homeless and unemployed, must be put on the political agenda, and the causes of their marginalisation – the operation of the labour and housing markets and the benefits system – must be addressed. Ken Roberts, more specifically, points to the need for a policy of full employment if education and training programmes are to be effective, and for non-manual unskilled jobs to be upgraded. In the context of the needs of young single mothers, Robert Page calls for effective education and training programmes, a good supply of affordable Local-Authority or housing-association accommodation, encouragement for young single mothers to stay in full-time education, a carer's allowance and state-provided child-care facilities. Related to Page's proposals, Helen Jones demands a national system of full-time nursery education for all children whose parents desire it. This broad agenda for action is an indication of how far Britain still has to go to create a classless society. The need for such an agenda is clear from the evidence of widespread poverty in Britain, a potent reminder of the continuing importance of class position in today's society.

One in three children now lives in a poor family according to the EU definition of poverty: that is, under half the national average income. Children of lone parents, who constitute about 19 per cent of families with dependent children, are especially at risk of poverty, as are certain ethnic minority children. Poverty among lone parents has risen in recent years; roughly 1 million lone parents are receiving income support, and this is expected to rise to 1.4 million by the end of the century. Although their need to work is greater, and many would like to work, lone parents actually find it harder to take up paid work: in the mid-1990s 39 per cent of lone mothers were employed compared with 62 per cent of married ones. The main policy directed at lone parents in recent years was the 1991 Child Support Act, which has financially disadvantaged more women than it has benefited (Millar 1996: 45, 47; Wasoff and Morris 1996: 68, 78).

The poverty of children is unevenly spread between ethnic groups, and so class-related inequalities are also racialised. Ethnic-minority children are more likely to be living in families on a low income and to experience high material and social deprivation. The Irish suffer the worst material and social deprivation of all groups and have the highest proportion of families on low incomes. Afro-Caribbeans also suffer high levels of deprivation (Oppenheim 1991). Only 34 per cent of children of Caribbean descent are living with a married couple, whereas 54 per cent are with a lone mother, and there is much evidence that families headed by a lone mother are especially vulnerable to poverty. For those in employment, average hourly full-time rates are as low as £4.78 for Pakistani and Bangladeshi women, compared with £6.59 for White women, and £6.87 for Pakistani and Bangladeshi men compared with £8.34 for Whites.

Asian children do better at GCSEs than all other groups, including Whites. At the age of 18, 65 per cent of Indians, 61 per cent of Pakistanis and Bangladeshis, 72 per cent of other Asians and 50 per cent of Black young people are still in full-time education, compared with 38 per cent of Whites, yet unemployment is much higher among all minority groups. Black, Pakistani and Bangladeshi people, in particular, have unemployment rates three times as high as Whites (*Guardian*, 8 August 1996). Those ethnic groups that are over-represented in the unemployment figures are often the groups that are least likely to claim their full state benefits. Problems with benefit agencies include a lack of multilingual facilities and discrimination due to racism and erroneous cultural assumptions (Law *et al.* 1996). Problems for children and young people living in poverty tend not to come singly but in multiples. These problems and their implications are examined in the following chapter.

REFERENCES

Crompton, R. (1993) *Class and Stratification: An Introduction to Current Debates*, Cambridge: Polity Press.

Blair, T. (1995) 'Power for a Purpose', *Renewal*, 3(4): 13.

Bourdieu, P. (1973) 'Cultural reproduction and social reproduction', in R.

Brown (ed.) *Knowledge, Education and Social Change*, London: Tavistock Publications.

Dahrendorf, R. (1959) *Class and Class Conflict in Industrial Society*, London: Routledge & Kegan Paul.

Edgell, S. (1993) *Class*, London: Routledge.

Ellis, N.W. (1991) *John Major: A Personal Biography*, London: Macdonald.

European Commission (1994) *Internal Market Current Status Community Social Policy*, 6, Luxembourg, 1 July.

Kelsall, K., Kelsall, H. and Chisholm, L. (1984) *Stratification*, London: Longman.

Law, I., Deacon, A., Hylton, C. and Karmani, A. (1996) 'Black families and social security: Evidence from fieldwork in Leeds', in H. Jones and J. Millar (eds) *The Politics of the Family*, Aldershot: Avebury.

Lockwood, D. (1958) *The Blackcoated Worker*, London: Unwin University Books.

Major, J. (1993) 'Conservatism in the 1990s: Our common purpose', Carlton Club Political Committee 1993 Lecture.

Miliband, R. (1989) *Divided Societies: Class Struggle in Contemporary Capitalism*, Oxford: Clarendon Press.

Millar, J. (1996) 'Poor mothers and absent fathers: Support for lone parents in comparative perspective', in H. Jones and J. Millar (eds) *The Politics of the Family*, Aldershot: Avebury.

Oppenheim, C. (1991) *Poverty in London: An Overview*, London: CPAG.

Townsend, P. (1992) *Hard Times*, Liverpool: Liverpool University Press.

Wasoff, F. and Morris, S. (1996) 'The Child Support Act: A victory for women?', in H. Jones and J. Millar (eds) *The Politics of the Family*, Aldershot: Avebury.

Chapter 2

Young people, class and poverty

Tony Novak

INTRODUCTION

Young people are not a homogeneous group. Despite the process of transition from young person to adult that they all have in common, and despite the aspirations to a universal 'youth culture', the experiences and life chances of young people, like those of their parents, differ greatly. A young upper-class person at public school in Leamington, waiting to go on to university and then to a more-or-less assured career in the civil service, finance or industry may experience similar anxieties about self-identity, sexuality and the other preoccupations of the young. But, in terms of material, educational and social advantage and security, the world such a person encounters is vastly different from that of the young working-class person on a Leeds or Liverpool housing estate.

That a tiny minority of young people, both now and in their adult lives, will never face the pressures of poverty is simply a matter of class. Although they themselves may not possess wealth or an income – although in reality many will have had trusts and other tax-saving devices set up for them by their parents – the certainty of a future inheritance offers them a present and future security that few ever dream of. Others, below the elevated ranks of the super-rich, are similarly protected by the stock of material, social and cultural capital – of money, educational opportunities, contacts and job opportunities – through which the middle classes pass on their advantage to subsequent generations (see, e.g., Allatt 1993; Roker 1993). For a large number of young people, however, both childhood and adolescence are often times of deprivation, while for the poorest they are times of significant harm to health, future prospects and general well-being.

The idea of a classless society flies in the face of this social reality. This reality, moreover, is one of increasing, rather than diminishing, inequality and polarisation. Whatever progress was made during the post-war era in reducing income and wealth differentials, in extending educational opportunities and in curbing class inequalities in health, housing, employment and unemployment, over the past two decades this progress has been firmly reversed. Poverty and growing class inequalities in the 1990s affect all age groups, but seem to bear especially heavily on children and the young. Their effects are to imprint upon a generation not only the material scars of poverty but also the social and individual consequences – among which must be counted the lowered self-esteem, the reduced expectations, the sense of insecurity, the lack of opportunity and fulfilment and the frustrations – that they are likely to carry forward into adult life.

Children are not normally seen as possessing an income or as having a class position in their own right. Inevitably, the poverty of children, like the wealth of children, is a reflection of that of their parents. As the rich have got richer – with the income of the top 10 per cent of households increasing by 61 per cent between 1979 and 1993 – the poor have got poorer, with the income of the poorest falling in real terms by 18 per cent over the same period (Department of Social Security 1995a). Of course, children bring an added financial burden to all parents, with the result that, other things being equal, standards of living in a household are likely to fall as children are born, until they leave and begin to earn their own living. Other things have not remained equal, however, and, as a result of both growing inequalities in employment and wages and declining levels of benefit, many families with children have found themselves increasingly poor. Currently, 3.7 million children – 29 per cent of all children – live on or below the state's minimal level of Income Support: an increase from 1.5 million in 1979 (Oppenheim and Harker 1996: 30). In relative terms, 33 per cent of children live at less than half the average income – over three times the proportion that did so in 1979. It is not only the case that large numbers of children are now more likely to experience poverty, but also that they are more likely to find themselves among the poorest. In 1979 half of the poorest households had children to support; by 1994 this had increased to two-thirds.

The effects of poverty on children are both deep and long-lasting, and are to be counted not only in terms of income, but also in terms of poorer health, increased risk of premature death, of accidents and injury, poorer housing, educational and recreational opportunities, greater stress, and the myriad other inequalities of social class. These effects of the early experience of poverty are compounded by the experience of adolescence and young adulthood. Young people of all classes face an often painful process of transition to adulthood, but the hardening of class differentials means that for many it is an experience of continuing poverty and prolonged dependence, of unemployment or low-waged and insecure work. The struggle to create and maintain a positive self-identity in these conditions is, moreover, made even more difficult by a Government policy that exacerbates the situation and treats many such young people with barely-disguised contempt.

GROWING UP POOR

The fact that one in three children are now growing up in households that have to survive on less than half of average income has enormous consequences not only for the present but also for the future. Poverty has many dimensions, but among them are its effects on health, which are both damaging and likely to be long-lasting. The Department of Health itself has recognised the obvious fact that 'the health of children is of major importance not only in its own right, but also as a determinant of adult health and of the health of the next generation' (cited Kumar 1993: 95). But Kumar's comprehensive review of the existing evidence and data on children and health shows that, in terms of both income and social class, poor children are twice as likely to die in infancy, are more susceptible to chronic and limiting illnesses, and have shorter lives as adults than their more affluent counterparts.

The full and cumulative effects of growing poverty in the 1980s and 1990s on the health of children have yet to be seen. Among young people the differential legacies of childhood are compounded in the growing inequalities of opportunity and experience of the young:

> Perhaps the biggest obstacle of all to understanding the health needs of young people has been the assumption that adolescence and health go hand in hand, what Bennett referred to as 'a widespread belief that they are a fit and healthy group'. This assumption, which still pervades much medical thinking, is rapidly being shaken by evidence concerning the health of young

people themselves and by a broader concern with the social and economic conditions they face as they enter adulthood. Economic recession, unemployment, low-paid jobs, and the sense of having no future are potentially all components of a social malaise that may affect the health of us all, but especially the young.

(West and Sweeting 1996: 50)

Like children, homeless young people are particularly vulnerable, and of these a large proportion are young working-class people who are estranged from their families or who have as children been in the care of a Local Authority. A survey of 16–26 year olds estranged from their families conducted by the National Children's Home (NCH) and published in *A Lost Generation?* in 1993 revealed disproportionate levels of physical and mental ill-health. Living on an average income of £34 each per week, nearly all had inadequate diets, two-thirds were in debt and half had considered resorting to shoplifting and theft to survive. According to the chief executive of NCH, 'the years between childhood and adulthood are supposedly the happiest years of your life. In stark contrast these teenagers are trapped in a lifestyle of poverty and deep despair'. (Cited the *Independent*, 9 November 1993).

This despair is counted most graphically in the rising rates of suicide, especially among young men. Having remained stable at around 65 per million from 1975 to 1984, the suicide rate for men aged 15–24 rose to 110 per million by 1990 (Wilkinson 1994: 39), although that for young women rose much more slowly, tempered by rising female employment and an increase in the birth rate to women under 20. What drives young men to take their own lives is inevitably a complex issue, and is not always related to social class and poverty, but a study of 1,000 young people from the west of Scotland, who were followed from the age of 15 to 21, found a significant deterioration in the mental health of those who became unemployed:

At 15 years remarkably little variation in health was found between respondents from different social class backgrounds. . . . However, the relationship of health to respondents' own economic position at the age of 18 presents a striking contrast. . . . For almost all the mental health measures, unemployed males and females were in poorer health. . . . Nine per cent of males and seven per cent of females who were unemployed reported attempting suicide, much higher rates than those found for those at work or in education.

(West and Sweeting 1996: 56/7)

The same factors that adversely affect the health of poor children and young people similarly limit their educational opportunities and achievement. As in health, fundamental inequalities of social class and income group survived the educational and other reforms of the post-war welfare state. The replacement of these structures – which at least aspired to some notion of greater equality – with social policies based on an explicit rejection of equality as a legitimate pursuit of Government policy has, since the 1980s, seen the educational divide widen again (Kumar 1993; Smith and Noble 1995). Again, as with health, the effects of class are felt both in the unequal start that people have and the unequal resources they receive. In a report on a primary school in one northern city that could be replicated in hundreds of other inner-city schools, Nick Davies noted how 'poverty invades the school':

> You can see it in the fabric of the building, which has bars on its windows and a spiked fence round its grounds. . . . It touches the physical well-being of the children, who sleep in damp houses and turn up wheezing; who wake up to find no food in the house and come to school crying with hunger – in such numbers that seven months ago the school started laying on breakfast. And it touches their personalities as they grow up in families which have collapsed under the weight of their hardship.
>
> (*Guardian*, 17 September 1995)

To the effects of poverty on children and young people themselves have now to be added the consequences of an increasingly divided and selective educational system, which in the name of 'choice' and 'diversity' offers the more affluent, the more articulate and the more powerful the opportunity to secure a better educational outcome for their children and, with that, a greater chance of future material prosperity and privilege. Meanwhile the poorest face declining and deteriorating schools, growing numbers of which, in their desperation to claw their way back up the 'league table' in order to attract more pupils and more money, deal with the problems that are created by excluding those – disproportionately Black pupils – that they find difficult to teach (Bridges 1994).

Once past school-leaving age, educational opportunities for working-class young people remain similarly restricted. Not only is university education often intimidating, if not unattainable, but restrictions on Local Authority spending have had particular impact on cuts in discretionary grants for day-release and further-education courses. For those who are unemployed, the opportunity to gain qualifications through part-time study has been further reduced through new restrictions on social security claimants and their availability for work (Unemployment Unit 1995).

EMPLOYMENT AND UNEMPLOYMENT

The need of young people to enter into paid employment always has been and remains differentiated according to social class. Traditionally, young people of the upper and middle classes have deferred entry into paid work through staying on at school, and by moving into further and higher education, in order to gain the qualifications that would provide them with entry to the higher reaches of the labour market. For young people of working-class origin the entry into paid work has traditionally come much earlier, as they have left – or been pushed off – the educational ladder to take up the jobs for which their class background has by and large determined them. The collapse of job opportunities for young people since the late 1970s has therefore affected some groups much more than others.

In the wake of this collapse the growth of youth training schemes and the expansion of further, and latterly of higher, education has failed substantially to alter inequalities of employment prospects among the young. The highly differentiated nature of this provision – from the barely-obscured cheap-labour 'training' schemes of stacking supermarket shelves on the one hand, through various forms of better-quality training and new vocational qualifications, to the expansion of university education on the other – simply replicated existing class divisions and opportunities. As Roberts (1993) points out, what upward social mobility for working-class youth there has been in the past fifteen years has been a reflection of the changing structure of the labour market and its expansion of skilled and professional jobs at the expense of unskilled jobs. But within this process, class differentials have remained:

> The same developments that have drawn more working-class young people up the educational and occupational ladders have simultaneously reduced the chances of middle-class children descending. . . . the relative inequalities in life chances, the greater likelihood of middle-class than working-class children reaching middle-class destinations, remained virtually unchanged.
>
> (Roberts 1993: 243)

What is more, those conditions that have allowed a degree of upward mobility for a minority of working-class young people have at the same time created a deterioration in the position of others:

> From a working-class perspective, an equally significant change in the 1980s was the increased risks of descent. Young people who failed to enter short careers and reasonably secure jobs stood real risks of unemployment and survival on poverty incomes with no escapes in sight. For certain groups of young people, the risks of long-term unemployment, or joblessness broken only by low-paid, short-lived jobs and schemes, were considerable.
>
> (Roberts 1993: 244)

For a substantial number of working-class young people the outlook in the 1990s is bleak. Trapped in a vicious circle of dead-end and low-paid work, inadequate Government training schemes or enforced unemployment, their poverty has become increasingly severe and visible. For those who do enter into paid employment, wage levels and conditions of work have deteriorated markedly. More than four times as many 16- to 24-year-old young men are in temporary jobs than any other age group, and only one-third have a union in their workplace (*Independent*, 25 September 1995). Prompted in part by an (ultimately futile and unsuccessful) Government policy intended to 'price' young people back into work – which saw, among other steps, the abolition in 1986 of Wages Council protection for young workers – wages for those under 18 fell from 42 per cent of adult rates in 1979 to 35 per cent by 1994; those for 18–20-year-olds from 61 per cent to 49 per cent (Low Pay Unit 1994: 9). By 1994, 46 per cent of 16-year-olds and 45 per cent of 17-year-olds in work were earning less than the National Insurance threshold: an increase from 10 per cent and 7 per cent respectively only four years earlier (Unemployment Unit 1995). Although low pay has become an increasing experience for many workers, its increase has become even more marked among the young:

> The relative fortunes of younger workers on low wages (i.e. those under 29) have deteriorated markedly since the late 1970s, from being almost 70 per cent of overall median earnings to just over half. . . . The relative pay of this group deteriorated faster than low-paid workers overall.
>
> (Research Findings 1994: 1)

While the earnings of young people as a whole have fallen relative to adults, class inequalities in earnings tend to be lower among younger workers than they are among older workers. This reflects the fact that the earnings of non-manual workers, and especially of managerial and professional groups, increase with age, while those of manual workers increase more slowly, reach a plateau, and often decline. Nevertheless, such inequalities are apparent. For workers under the age of 18 there are no comparative data, since very few upper- or middle-class young people enter employment at this age; the vast majority of those who do are unskilled manual workers. At the age of 20 earnings are roughly equal between manual and non-manual workers, but by the age of 24 non-manual workers are beginning to earn more: 15 per cent more in the case of young men, and 29 per cent more in the case of young women. Within particular occupational groups, the differences are more marked. A young woman in her early twenties earns on average 61 per cent more in a professional occupation than in a sales or clerical occupation, while a similar male administrator or manager earns 41 per cent more than his counterpart in 'other' – unclassified – occupations (Department of Employment 1994).

However, at least until young people reach their twenties, employment remains a minority destination. Those who do enter the labour market face a situation in which, since the late 1970s, employers have not only been able to be highly selective but have actively discriminated against particular groups of the young. Once 'the conventional pool of young recruits has been exhausted, employers have turned to older workers and women returners rather than, for example, young people from ethnic minorities or those with few formal qualifications, who are too often vulnerable to stereotypical assumptions about their attitudes to work and personal characteristics' (Williamson 1993: 34). The result is that unemployment – already disproportionately higher for young people than for other age groups – is particularly concentrated among the least qualified and (despite their qualifications) among ethnic minorities. Thus a recent Labour Force Survey estimates that 62 per cent of Black young men in London aged 16–24 were unemployed – three times the rate for White young men – while the youth unemployment rate in inner-city Manchester, Liverpool and London is six times higher than in mid-Sussex (*Independent*, 20 November 1995).

Official unemployment statistics count only those unemployed who claim benefit, and so have excluded most 16- and 17-year-olds since they were barred from receiving benefit in 1988. Yet the Labour Force survey shows that one in five of this age group were not in education or training or employment. Despite a fall of 11 per cent in the number of young people as a whole between 1990 and 1994, and a rise in the numbers staying on in education, among 18–24 year olds unemployment rose by a third to over 615,000, while their rate of unemployment doubled from 9 to 18 per cent (Unemployment Unit 1995). At the beginning of 1996 the unemployment rate for 18- and 19-year-olds was twice as high as the national average, and over 50 per cent higher for 20–24-year-olds (Department of Employment 1996). Over the period from 1990 to 1994 the proportion of young people unemployed for twelve months or more increased from 16 to 24 per cent (Unemployment Unit 1994). By 1996 it was still at this level: out of over half a million unemployed 19–24-year-olds, 136,000 had been out of work for between six and twelve months, and 130,000 for over a year (Department of Employment 1996). For those unemployed, and especially for those unemployed for long periods of time, changes made to the state benefit system for young people have had a particularly severe effect.

BENEFITS

The depression of young people's expectations – and especially those of young working-class people – that was a hallmark, even a target, of Government policy from 1979 was given expression through the changing benefit regime for young people. In part, policy reflected particular concerns about the young: their disproportionately high levels of unemployment, the apparent unwillingness of employers to take on young people, and the by no means new preoccupation with alienated or challenging youth. In part, it reflected a wider Government strategy towards the poor in general, aimed at undermining welfare entitlements, reducing state responsibility and reasserting the financial and moral responsibilities of families, whatever the cost to families and young people themselves. In consequence, many young people found themselves stripped of entitlement to benefit, subject to increasing regulation and monitoring, and faced with a redefinition of adulthood within the social security system that would in most cases deny them the status of adults until the age of 25.

Not surprisingly these changes had the greatest impact on working-class young people, and especially on the poorest, who were more likely to be in need of state support. Starting in 1980, with the abolition of supplementary benefit to school-leavers until the start of the next academic term, progressive restrictions were imposed on young people's entitlement to housing benefit, board and lodgings payments and other benefits, while tighter regulations were imposed on their availability for work and their ability to engage in part-time education. By 1987, fourteen significant changes had been made to young people's entitlements, at a total cost to young people of £200 million (Andrews and Jacobs 1990: 77). The 1988 Social Security Act finally abolished Income Support entitlement for all but a tightly-prescribed group of 16- and 17-year-olds, and introduced a lower rate of benefit for single claimants under the age of 25.

Although Andrews and Jacobs argue that 'it is hard to escape the conclusion that the young have been deliberately selected as easy targets in the assault against benefits' (ibid.: 74) it is clear that the ease of targeting young people has not been the only consideration. As *The Times* noted in 1983, the targeting of young people's benefits, while 'primarily to allow the DHSS to offer a meaty sacrifice on the altar of the Public Expenditure Survey Committee . . . [is] also, more important for the long run, to establish the violability of basic social benefits and do it for a group over which the political screams will not be too loud' (cited in Allbeson 1985: 86). Since then basic social benefits once considered inviolable, not only for the young but also for the rest of the poor, have been subject to increasing cutbacks and restrictions. Allied to tax cuts for the more affluent, this has made state policy a more significant factor in the increasing inequality and division in society than changes in the labour market, including the growth of unemployment and low-paid work. Britain by the mid-1990s had become a more unequal society than at any time in its history, and continued to become more unequal at a rate unparalleled in the rest of the world, with the sole exception of New Zealand.

Within this trajectory of increasing inequality, the fate of young people is especially significant. As the future generation of adults, parents and workers, their experience is crucial in determining what will or will not be considered as acceptable, or at least unchallengeable in the future. In this sense, the assault on young people has spearheaded an assault on a generation that has become the target for the imposition of new work disciplines, lower expectations in terms of both social security benefits and job security, pay and conditions, and a sexual, social and moral agenda that the New Right under the governments of both Thatcher and Major has pursued in the face of both uncertain evidence and immense hardship to some of the most vulnerable of the young.

The reinforcement of work discipline has, since its origins, been a major preoccupation of the social security system (Novak 1988). This has been particularly true in times of high unemployment, when the state's role in maintaining 'work incentives' has had to compensate for the lack of work available. It has also, and especially at such times, embodied a major preoccupation with the young. The disciplining of young people to the world of work, especially to the constraints and monotonies that characterise the job opportunities of many working-class youth, has always been a problem. Young people often lack the responsibilities and commitments of parenthood or mortgages, and the curbing of their enthusiasm and rebelliousness has required a mass of social, cultural and economic constraints. When, as is currently the case, even poorly-paid and dead-end jobs are in short supply, the problem of disciplining young people, both as young people and as the next generation of adults, becomes more acute.

Throughout the 1980s Government thinking on the young unemployed was influenced by the belief that young people had not only 'priced themselves out of work' through their wage expectations but had also excluded themselves through their negative attitudes towards employers and the employment they offered, their refusal to accept arbitrary authority and discipline, and their supposed preference for an easy life on benefit. When the Conservative election manifesto in 1987 announced that it would take steps 'to ensure that those under eighteen who deliberately choose to remain unemployed are not eligible for benefit' (cited in Andrews and Jacobs 1990: 79) it confirmed the trend towards compulsory training as the only allowable option for the young unemployed. The question of whether young people 'chose' to remain unemployed – or whether their unemployment was a product of an inadequate labour market or inefficient and unpopular training schemes – was simply ignored in the decision to abolish entitlement to benefit for all those under 18. Since then 16- and 17-year-olds unable to find a job or a place on a training scheme and without families (or with families that are unable or unwilling to support them) have formed a growing number of the destitute and homeless. In 1994, 97,000 16–17-year-olds had no work and no training place, and of these only 28,000 received any income, mostly in the form of the tightly controlled Severe Hardship Allowance – which is payable only to those who are at serious risk of abuse or of significant harm to their health (Unemployment Unit 1994). One survey of young people who had claimed this allowance, conducted by the Coalition on Young People and Social Security in the early 1990s, found that 45 per cent had been or still were homeless, and half had no money; a quarter said that they had had to beg, steal or sell drugs in order to survive, a quarter already had criminal convictions, and a quarter of the girls were pregnant (cited Wilkinson 1994: 36). For a number of young people, the lack of a supportive family and of any prospect of employment has been met by a state policy which, in denying them benefit, has turned them into outcasts, vulnerable to the most damaging exploitation:

> Home Office figures show that between 1989 and 1993 nearly 1,500 young people under 18 were convicted of offences relating to prostitution and a further 1,800 were cautioned. The numbers are rising. . . . According to the Chief Executive of the Church of England charity the Children's Society, 'prostitution is very often a survival strategy for young people on the streets who have no money, food or shelter'.
>
> (*Guardian*, 18 October 1995)

Those over 18 have fared little better. The poverty of a large number of young people is reflected in the fact that, despite numerous disqualifications from benefit, 894,000 men and 811,000 women under the age of 30 were entitled to claim means-tested Income Support in May 1994. This included an increase in single male claimants from 426,000 in 1989 to 751,000 by 1994, and in single female claimants from 604,000 to 794,000 (Department of Social Security 1995b: 22). The decision in 1988 to pay a reduced rate of benefit to single claimants under the age of 25 – with the result that those over 25 receive 28 per cent more benefit, before housing costs, than those under 25 – was based on an argument that the majority of 18–25 year olds were not themselves householders, and that all therefore should be treated as dependents. This was despite the fact that, even under the constrained benefit regime of the time, half of all claimants between the ages of 21 and 24, and one-third of those age between 18 and 24, lived as independent adults. Whether this reduction in benefit was successful in throwing young people back onto the resources of their parents, or whether it merely intensified the poverty that they faced as young adults, makes little difference.

As with adults, the payment of benefit to most young people remains conditional upon their being available for work. Over the past decade, the interpretation and test of this availability, and the sanctions imposed for failing to meet it, have been extended, culminating in the introduction of the Jobseeker's Allowance in 1996. Insofar as it affects young people, this legislation maintains the exclusion from benefit of most 16–17-year-olds, and replaces Unemployment Benefit for those who have previously contributed to the scheme with a maximum of six months (rather than twelve months) benefit set at the lower rate of Income Support. Like the Income Support for the uninsured unemployed, which it also replaces, the Jobseeker's Allowance has introduced a lower rate of benefit for all single claimants under the age of 25, whether they have paid insurance contributions or not. Set at one quarter of the average starting salary of 16-year-olds, this level of benefit properly reflects 'the lower earnings expectation of people in that group', according to the Secretary of State for Social Security (cited in the *Financial Times*, 27 January 1994). As a result, a quarter of young men and over a third of young women previously eligible for Unemployment Benefit found their income reduced by 20 per cent (Department of Social Security 1995b: 156).

But it is not only in the level of the new benefit but also in the conditions attached to it that the Government's intentions are made clear. Described by the Conservative Research Department (cited in the *Guardian* 17 January 1996) as introducing a series of 'sanctions on the workshy', the Jobseeker's Act gives new and wide-ranging powers to officials 'to direct jobseekers to improve their employability through, for example, attending a course to improve jobseeking skills or motivation, or taking steps to present themselves acceptably to employers' (cited Finn and Murray 1995: 310), on pain of being suspended from benefit. The interpretation of who is 'acceptable' to employers, and on what terms, widens significantly the scope of the discretionary powers used by officials in their dealings with so-called 'new-age travellers', Black claimants and other young people whose appearance or attitudes may conflict with that considered appropriate, and it further extends the scope – already

well-documented (see NACAB 1991; Cooper 1985; Amin 1992) –
for bias and discrimination against particular groups.

YOUNG MOTHERS

The spectre of a generation of wilfully unemployed, idle young
people scorning the world of work and content to live off the state
may bear little relation to the reality of young people's lives and
aspirations (Holman 1994/5), but fuels a state policy that, in the
absence of meaningful opportunities for employment, consistently
penalises those that are its victims. A similar process is also established in dealing with the other great spectre that hovered over
Conservative Party conferences during the first half of the 1990s:
the supposed growing legions of single young women choosing to
have babies. Class distinctions in the perception of and response to
illegitimacy have always reflected that dual standard which distinguishes the experience of women of independent financial means –
of whom Sarah Keyes, mistress of former Conservative Party
chairman Cecil, now Lord, Parkinson and mother of his illegitimate
child, is but one example – from that of those single women for
whom motherhood means dependence on the state, whether they
wish it or not. To this has been added a new moral panic centred on
right-wing fears of the decline of marriage and the family and, in
particular, on the erosion of the role and authority of fathers.
Paradoxically, this revival of Victorian paternalism, with its backlash against the provision of sex education and birth control for
young people, and its attempts to limit state support for unmarried
young mothers, can be seen to have exacerbated the problem for
young people, rather than helping solve it (Selman and Glendinning
1994/5).

The imagery of single parenthood that has dominated public
discussion of the issue through the first half of the 1990s barely
conceals the class bias of its vision of young, often teenage and
uneducated, working-class girls choosing to live off the state.
Although the reality of this situation is far more complex, as the
following chapters show, this imagery has significantly informed
state policies towards this group. Such examples mirror the state's
response to young unemployed men and women in penalising the
poorest and most vulnerable. In a class-structured society it has
always been thus, but during the 1990s the claims of a classless
society have sat uneasily alongside a new vocabulary for describing

the poor and a marked shift in policy that have further isolated the poor and justified their neglect.

AN UNDERCLASS

It is – at least at first sight – a major irony of a so-called 'classless society' that the 1990s have seen politicians, media commentators and policy-makers direct growing attention on what has come to be known as an 'underclass'. Much of this attention has focused on the young, or at least on certain groups of working-class youth who are Black, unemployed or single mothers and who are depicted as flouting the norms and rules of civilised society. In response, state policy has adopted an increasingly strident and intolerant tone towards them. Rather than address the fundamental problems of poverty and inequality and their consequences, policy has shifted towards punishment, containment and control. In this process, attempts to understand and explain the complexity of the problems facing many working-class young people have been abandoned, often to be replaced by simple labels of 'bad' or 'evil' that place the blame for their situation on young people themselves.

For the most part, those who have argued that poverty in Britain in the 1990s is taking a new and threatening form in the shape of an 'underclass' have focused their attention on what they see as the distinctive (and abnormal) behaviour, values and attitudes of particular groups of the poor. Thus, according to Charles Murray – a leading American right-wing theorist sponsored by the *Sunday Times* to report on the emergence of an 'underclass' in Britain – ' "underclass" does not refer to degree of poverty, but to a type of poverty . . . [they are] defined by their behaviour' (Murray 1990: 1). This behaviour – supposedly evidenced in welfare dependence, the rejection of the work ethic, of marriage and of the nuclear family, and in the growth of long-term unemployment and criminal activity – is seen as 'a plague . . . whose values are now contaminating entire neighbourhoods' (Murray 1990: 3–4), and whose spread threatens to engulf the whole of society.

Central to Murray's argument is the view that it is the laxity of social welfare, the absence of punishment for offenders, and the benefits made available (especially to the young working class) in the form of access to housing, unemployment and other benefits that was responsible for creating this situation:

In the 1960s and 1970s social policy in Britain fundamentally changed what makes sense. The changes did not affect the mature as much as the young. They affected the affluent hardly at all. Rather, the rules of the game changed fundamentally for low-income young people. Behaviour changed along with the rules.

(Murray 1990: 25)

This change in the rules – which meant that, for the poor, single motherhood 'went from "extremely punishing" to "not so bad" ' (Murray 1990: 30) – is held responsible for the rise in illegitimacy: 'the best predictor of an underclass in the making' (Murray 1990: 4). With this, it is argued, came a collapse in the social fabric of poor communities. According to the *Sunday Times*:

The past two decades have witnessed the growth of whole communities in which the dominant family structure is the single-parent on welfare, whose male offspring are already immersed in a criminal culture by the time they are teenagers and whose daughters are destined to follow in the family tradition of unmarried teenage mothers. It is not just a question of a few families without fathers; it is a matter of whole communities with barely a single worthwhile male role-model. No wonder the youths of the underclass are uncontrollable by the time (sometimes before) they are teenagers. . . . In communities without fathers, the overwhelming evidence is that youngsters begin by running wild and end up running foul of the law.

(*Sunday Times*, 28 February 1993)

This 'overwhelming evidence', however, is by no means so clear-cut. Undeniably there are major changes taking place in Britain in the 1990s, not all of them for the better, but not all of them for the worse. The increase in violence, the growth of poverty, inequality and social polarisation, the breakdown and discrediting of the law and the challenge to male superiority and dominance have all contributed to a sense of unease and crisis. But these changes are not confined to poor communities, still less can they be clearly seen as the consequences of the attitudes and behaviour of the poor themselves. Indeed, a substantial amount of research into the attitudes and values of the so-called 'underclass' reveals a remarkable attachment to the dominant values of hard work, independence, respect for the law and the family (see, e.g., Smith 1992; Brown 1990; Payne and Payne 1994; Gallie 1994).

Nevertheless, the concept of the 'underclass' continues to have political purchase and to inform state policy towards the young. In their pronouncements on young single mothers, Government ministers, such as the Home Secretary Michael Howard, have blamed them for the fact that 'children, instead of learning the difference between right and wrong, instead concentrate on how not to get caught' (*Independent*, 20 November 1993), while as Secretary of State for Wales, John Redwood argued that there was a widespread belief among the young that 'the illegitimate child is the passport to a council flat and a benefit income' (*Independent*, 14 August 1995). It is an image that is as little related to the realities of single parenthood as the effects of the Government's response are limited to those single mothers on whom the image is based. The ill-defined concept of 'the underclass' is such an elastic one that, especially in its application, it is capable of throwing its net over a much wider range of people. It was on the back of this image that the Government took steps in the 1996 Housing Act to end the automatic right not only of single mothers but also of other priority homeless groups to permanent Local Authority housing, replacing it instead with the offer only of temporary accommodation.

'The underclass', described by Kenneth Clarke (cited in the *Financial Times*, 7 December 1992) as 'the most formidable challenge facing western societies', has been depicted as the growth, especially among the young, of an alien and threatening culture that will not disappear even with the return of full employment or the restoration of meaningful opportunities. As the Labour MP Frank Field has argued:

> We've got a number of young people who are now outside the labour market, who've created their own world, partly through drugs, partly through crime, partly through drawing welfare, and who are not prepared to join Great Britain Ltd again on the terms that we offer. . . . That group is different from the vast majority of the unemployed, most of whom are anxious to return to work, almost on any terms.
>
> (BBC Radio 4, *Analysis*, 3 December 1992)

The policy implications of such a view are considerable, pointing as they do to a belief that the so-called 'underclass' will not respond to the ordinary measures and incentives – 'the terms that we offer' – and that more drastic, and if necessary punitive, action will be required. This has already become evident in the introduction of the

Jobseeker's Allowance, which the Labour opposition in 1996 declined to undertake to abolish, should it come to power. It is also most strikingly evident in the practices of the criminal justice system. Arguing that 'what many commentators refer to as "the underclass" – a class that is beneath the working class' was to be found in places 'where unemployed youths – often Black youths – congregate', the Metropolitan Police Commissioner took the view that the policing of such communities, with their evident disrespect for the law, could not have 'an over-regard for individual liberties' (cited Campbell 1993: 108). The result was the adoption of 'swamp' operations and military-style policing, especially of Black communities and Black youth, with consequent injuries and fatalities and increased tensions between the police and the communities they were meant to serve.

Black youth has not figured predominantly in the literature on the 'underclass' in Britain compared to the USA, where it is seen as an overwhelmingly Black phenomenon. According to Charles Murray, for example, the Black population in Britain is too small to have a significant independent effect. Nevertheless, in terms of policy and the state's response to young people, Black youth figures highly, especially (as later chapters will show) in such areas as criminal justice policy, school exclusions and children and young people in care. As implementation of these areas of policy becomes more unrelenting and punitive, so those at the receiving end have their alienation and sense of abandonment by the state even further confirmed.

This shift in policy, predicated on a view of 'the underclass', has had the effect of further reinforcing both the image and the position of such young people as a group at the margins of society. As Williamson, among others, has argued, state policy towards young people – and in particular towards the poorest and most disadvantaged – was, even for a large part of the 1980s, based on a view that all young people, if given sufficient opportunity, had a positive contribution to make towards society:

> Early state interventions remained based, to some extent at least, on dialogue and consultation, and policy initiatives retained some "social engineering" objectives which had been central to youth policy developments in the 1960s, in intent if not in practice. Increasingly, however, such objectives evaporated or were abandoned, replaced by dogmatic ideology which bore little relation to the realities of young people's lives or contemporary

social relationships. Youth policy development in the United Kingdom is steadily confirming the marginality of increasing proportions of certain groups of young people, and – although it is difficult to disentangle the differential effects of class, race and gender – policy has impinged most detrimentally on young people who are black, female, poorly qualified, with disabilities, from 'broken homes' and with criminal careers.

(Williamson 1993: 35)

CLASSLESS 'COMMONSENSE'

During the 1980s youth policy, like most other areas of state policy, was involved in a battle of both ideas and practice, as the social-democratic perspective which had dominated welfare provision since the 1950s came under repeated challenge from the political forces of the New Right. In part, this battle was one of backstage manoeuvring, as those who worked most closely with young people – teachers, social workers, probation officers and youth workers – fought to maintain the positive aspects of their work against cut-backs in resources and restrictions on their autonomy and areas of work. But the battle moved increasingly into the public arena, as ministers and politicians, both prompted and backed by the media, began publicly to denigrate the activities of those working within the welfare state and with young people, to ridicule and dismiss the theories and models from which they worked, and to put forward alternative and much more simplistic explanations of social issues and problems that would justify an increasingly coercive tilt in state policy.

Shortly after John Major's election as leader of the Conservative Party and as Prime Minister, his announcement of a 'Back to Basics' campaign exemplified this trend. Although this was temporarily derailed by a succession of sexual and financial scandals among members of his own Government, the significance of this campaign was not that it asserted a personal morality (which Government ministers were incapable of living up to) but that it asserted the primacy of a populist and simplistic 'common sense' over the need for the detailed research into, and explanations of, social issues and problems that had previously underpinned state policy. Rising levels of juvenile crime were not to be understood in the context of increasing poverty and inequality, or of the stresses and alienation of young people, but as a result of wickedness and the breakdown of respect for authority. The much-publicised growth of teenage unmarried motherhood was similarly to be blamed on the supposed liberality of state benefits and housing policies, while continuing high levels of youth unemployment were taken as confirmation of the existence of a lax dependency culture.

Behind such simplistic explanations lay a more-or-less conscious anti-intellectualism and a rejection of alternative attempts to understand and explain these events. The Downing Street Policy Unit briefing paper which launched the 'Back to Basics' campaign (*Sunday Times*, 5 November 1993) thus spoke of the need to challenge 'a number of social orthodoxies that took root in the 1960s'. Of particular concern were 'those areas of social policy where theorists dragged professionals and administrators furthest from common sense'. This attack on 'the trendy and shallow fashions of progressive opinion', which undoubtedly over-estimated the impact of left-wing theory and denied the validity of the knowledge and experience gained by those working within various areas of social policy, also reflected a long-standing preoccupation of the New Right with countering the influence of welfare professionals and other state administrators. Its translation into policy, however, has ushered in a series of changes with far-reaching and damaging consequences that have also provoked concern and resistance from within the state establishment itself.

This has been most plainly evident in the area of penal policy. In a key article in the *Guardian* (11 November 1993) David Faulkner, Deputy Secretary at the Home Office in charge of criminal justice policy until 1992, wrote of the Government's change of direction as:

> probably the most sudden and the most radical which has ever taken place in this area of public policy. Within a period of less than 12 months, much of [this] programme has been politically discredited and seems to have been largely abandoned. Overwhelming emphasis is now being placed on criminalisation, detection, conviction and punishment as the means of dealing not only with violence and other forms of serious crime, but also with what has previously been regarded (not always universally) as anti-social behaviour, for example squatting or interference with fox-hunting.

In defiance of overwhelming research and evidence that 'prison does not work' in reducing crime, successive measures have been introduced to stiffen the penalties for young offenders. Alongside this has gone a continuing portrayal of young offenders as wicked and wilfully anti-social. John Redwood, then Secretary of State for Wales, who had earlier achieved notoriety for his criticism of single mothers, thus spoke to a meeting of Welsh businessmen:

> The idea that the yobs who do these things have no choice, that they are creatures of circumstances, is nonsense. . . . Let us not call them probation service clients, disadvantaged youngsters or young offenders. Let us call them thieves, vandals and hooligans.
>
> (Cited in the *Financial Times*, 19 October 1993)

This demonisation of young offenders has been paralleled in governments' dealings with other groups of working-class youth. Across the spectrum, state policy has become more abrasive and unyielding. Following John Major's exhortation to 'condemn a little more, and understand a little less', rehabilitation has been pushed aside in favour of punishment and retribution; young people whose behaviour causes problems for schools have been simply excluded; the young unemployed have been further impoverished and subjected to more pressure and regulation; and those in work face growing insecurity, fewer rights and less pay. The policy changes that have resulted from this have simply served to marginalise disadvantaged young people even further, to deepen their poverty and to increase their sense of frustration and exclusion. As a result, the Conservatives increased the divide between the most disadvantaged and other young people. As Williamson reminds us:

> It is, of course, important to reiterate that more fortunate [sic] young people, with supportive family networks, find themselves propelled onto a more constructive path, whereby educational achievement opens doors to better quality training and employment futures, which in turn provide the resources to find routes into restricted housing markets, and thereby to personal, social and financial independence. For a growing minority of young people, however, the process of transition is both destructive and debilitating.
>
> (Williamson 1993: 43)

It is, however, not so much fortune as social class which determines whether a young person will be able to proceed to personal, social and financial independence. Growing inequalities of social class, affecting the young at least as much as everyone else, have over the past two decades come to challenge not only the idea of a classless society, but the very legitimacy of a society that allows, and indeed encourages, this growth in inequality. It is in defence of this situation that the labelling of significant groups as an incorrigible and self-destructive 'underclass' makes political sense. The apparent irony of an 'underclass' in the midst of a classless society serves to obscure the realities of class division (Levitas 1996). If we are to see ourselves as a classless society, then the abundant and growing evidence of class inequalities, their destructive impact on the lives, opportunities and aspirations of many of the young, and the moments of defiance or frustration that this provokes, needs to be hidden under a rhetoric that blames members of the so-called 'underclass' for their situation and justifies their neglect or punishment on the ground that they are not a part and product of society but a class outside it.

REFERENCES

Allatt, P. (1993) 'Becoming privileged: The role of family processes', in I. Bates and G. Riseborough *Youth and Inequality*, Buckingham: Open University Press.

Allbeson, J. (1985) 'Seen but not heard: Young people', in S. Ward (ed.) *DHSS In Crisis*, London: Child Poverty Action Group.

Amin, K. (1992) *Poverty in Black and White*, London: Child Poverty Action Group.

Andrews, K. and Jacobs J. (1990) *Punishing the Poor: Poverty Under Thatcher*, London: Macmillan.

Bridges, L. (1994) 'Tory education: Exclusion and the black child', *Race and Class* 36(1): 33–49.

Brown, C (1990) 'The focus on single mothers', in C. Murray *The Emerging British Underclass*, London: Institute of Economic Affairs.

Campbell, B. (1993) *Goliath: Britain's Dangerous Places*, London: Methuen.

Cooper, S. (1985) *Observations in Supplementary Benefit Offices*, London: Policy Studies Institute.

Department of Employment (1994) *New Earnings Survey*, London: HMSO.

—— (1996) *Labour Market Trends, June 1996*, London: HMSO.

Department of Social Security (1995a) *Households Below Average Income*, London: HMSO.

—— (1995b) *Social Security Statistics*, London: HMSO.

Finn, D. and Murray I. (1995) *Unemployment and Training Rights Handbook*, London: Unemployment Unit.

Gallie, D. (1994) 'Are the unemployed an underclass? Some evidence from the social change and economic life initiative', *Sociology* 28(3): 737–57.

Holman, B. (1994/5) 'Urban youth – Not an underclass', *Youth and Policy* 47: 69–77.

Kumar, V. (1993) *Poverty and Inequality in the UK: The Effects on Children*, London: National Children's Bureau.

Levitas, R. (1996) 'The concept of social exclusion and the new Durkheimian hegemony', *Critical Social Policy* 16(1): 5–20.

Low Pay Unit (1994) 'Whose economic upturn?' *New Review*, Nov/Dec: 6–9.

Murray, C. (1990) *The Emerging British Underclass*, London: Institute of Economic Affairs.

NACAB (1991) *Barriers to Benefit: Black Claimants and Social Security*, London: National Association of Citizens Advice Bureaux.

National Children's Home (1993) *A Lost Generation?: A Survey of the Problems faced by Vulnerable Young People Living on Their Own*, London: NCH.

Novak, T. (1988) *Poverty and the State: An Historical Sociology*, Milton Keynes: Open University Press.

Oppenheim, C. and Harker, L. (1996) *Poverty the Facts*, London: Child Poverty Action Group.

Payne, J. and Payne C. (1994) 'Recession, restructuring and the fate of the unemployed: Evidence in the underclass debate', *Sociology* 28(1): 1–19.

Research Findings (1994) No 52, York: Joseph Rowntree Foundation.

Roberts, K. (1993) 'Career trajectories and the mirage of increased social mobility', in I. Bates and G. Riseborough *Youth and Inequality*, Milton Keynes: Open University Press.

Roker, D. (1993) 'Gaining the edge: Girls at a private school', in I. Bates and G. Riseborough *Youth and Inequality*, Milton Keynes: Open University Press.

Selman, P. and Glendinning, C. (1994/5) 'Teenage parenthood and social policy', *Youth and Policy* 47: 39–58.

Smith, D. (ed.) (1992) *Understanding the Underclass,* London: Policy Studies Institute.

Smith, T. and Noble, M. (1995) *Education Divides: Poverty and Schooling in the 1990s*, London: Child Poverty Action Group.

Unemployment Unit (1994) *Working Brief*, 52, London: Unemployment Unit.

—— (1995) *Working Brief*, 63, London: Unemployment Unit.

West, P. and Sweeting, H. (1996) 'Nae job, nae future: Young people and health in a context of unemployment', *Health and Social Care in the Community* 4(1): 50–62.

Wilkinson, G. (1994) *Unfair Shares: The Effects of Widening Income Differentials on the Young*, Ilford: Barnardos.

Williamson, H. (1993) 'Youth policy in the United Kingdom and the marginalisation of young people', *Youth and Policy* 40: 33–48.

Chapter 3

The right start
Poverty, health and education

Helen Jones

INTRODUCTION

A classless society would be one in which class was no longer a significant variable in a person's life chances. This chapter reviews the wealth of evidence which demonstrates the continuing link between class position and standards of health among children and young people: the poorer the child, the poorer her or his health. Poverty increases the chances of poor health and low educational achievement in children, which in turn reduces their prospects of employment and decent wages. As it is the poverty and inequality which causes the poorer health, and not the ill-health which leads to poverty and inequality, it is the poverty and inequality which needs to be addressed first and foremost.

A broad-based strategy is required which goes beyond health policy. The call for such a strategy is nothing new; for instance, in 1979 the Black Report on *Inequalities in Health* demanded higher levels of child benefit and benefit for older children, an increased maternity grant, the introduction of an infant care allowance, free school meals for all children and more government investment in housing, as well as health-specific policies. These calls fell on stony ground (Townsend and Davidson 1982: 203–5).

This chapter argues the case for a comprehensive, high-quality national system of nursery education for all 3–5-year-olds whose parents desire it. This would be a means of offering parents the opportunity to seek paid work, and so pull the family out of poverty and off benefits, and would attack the link between poverty and ill-health. It would also be a means of giving all children a good start in the education system when they begin compulsory schooling at the age of 5; this good start can then be built on in order to help break the link between class position and educational attainment. Of course, this is not a panacea for all class-related inequalities, but a comprehensive system of nursery education would make an important contribution, at a cost which is within the bounds of political possibility. The drawback with most solutions to poverty and class inequalities is that they involve governments undertaking redistributions of resources so massive that they are not politically feasible; the problem therefore remains unresolved, and the close link between class inequalities and the health and well-being of children and young people continues.

One of the starkest facts that denies the hope that we may be moving towards a classless society is the growth in, and extensiveness of, poverty, especially among children. High unemployment, low wages, insecure employment, the absence of a comprehensive system of nursery schools (which would enable more mothers to enter the labour market and poorer children to start school in pole position), the absence or irrelevance of social policies to tackle child poverty, fiscal policies and the expansion in the numbers of lone parents have all contributed to the growth in child poverty. Youth poverty has also grown due to unemployment, the failure of Youth Training Schemes to guarantee a place for all young people, 16- and 17-year-olds' ineligibility for benefits and the lack of decent, affordable housing for them.

If we are assessing the prospects for reducing class inequalities in standards of health for the next generation, it is vital to consider the links between poverty, inequality and ill-health, and to take into account the current class-related patterns of health among children and young people. The effects of poverty can clearly be seen in the health of children.

CHILDREN'S AND YOUNG PEOPLE'S HEALTH

The health prospects for the next generation depend on the current health of infants and children (Power *et al.* 1990: 17–28). Links, for instance, have been detected between babies with low birth weight and health problems when they grow up (Barker *et al.* 1989: 577–80). In 1993 the Chief Medical Officer argued that establishing a healthy lifestyle during adolescence has a range of benefits: in the short-term a healthy lifestyle encourages optimum growth and resistance to physical and emotional ill-health, and in the long-term a healthy lifestyle in adulthood is more likely if it is established in youth

(Department of Health 1994). Standards of children's health are improving: death rates in infants and children are better than for any other age group. Children have fewer infections, they are taller and have better teeth than ever before. Overall improvements in standards of health should not detract, however, from the continuing class-related standards of health among children and young people.

The socio-economic environment into which a child is born has an immediate impact on its life chances. Over the years, research has shown a relationship between stillbirths and the perinatal and infant mortality rate, which in turn is related to socio-economic factors. To give one example from a recent piece of research, researchers looking into the high perinatal and neonatal mortality rate of UK-born Pakistani babies concluded that it was probably due to socio-economic factors (Bundey *et al.* 1991: 101–14).

It is generally agreed that breast-feeding provides the best start in life for children, and, here again, class inequalities are present. A mother is more likely to breast-feed if she is educated beyond the age of 18, if she is aged 25 or over, if she is from a higher class, if she lives in London and the south-east of England, if she is a non-smoker, and if the baby is one of her first (Department of Health 1990).

Growth is an important measure of health in children, and this has been found to correspond with children's class. Children in larger families and in families where the father is in a manual occupation or unemployed are likely to be shorter. Poverty and height are often linked: families on state benefits and with children receiving free school meals are likely to have shorter children. Inner-city children are also shorter. Socially deprived ethnic-minority children, however, show greater variation in their height, and Afro-Caribbean children tend to be taller than average. Smoking is now a class-related activity, and smoking in pregnancy correlates with lower-birth-weight babies and with shorter height in childhood. Children whose mothers smoked when they were pregnant, and whose parents continue to smoke, also tend to be shorter; they are also more likely to suffer from respiratory complaints (Department of Health 1990). Respiratory and gastro-intestinal infections are more common in poor families. Poor children are also worse affected by common childhood illnesses. Tooth decay among children is more widespread in industrial centres and among the poorer social classes.

A number of studies have continued to link poverty with poor diets. The School Milk Campaign found poor nutrition and poor growth rates among children from low income families. Malnutrition is seen as stunting growth and mental development. Dr Tony Waterston, convenor of the British Association for Community Child Health, told the press that the long-term effects of malnutrition are devastating for health, and it increases both behavioural problems among children and abuse from stressed parents. The Government's own Low Income Project Team, set up in June 1994 to review the evidence on diet, low income and ill-health, found evidence of malnutrition, although it was forbidden as part of its remit to discuss income-support levels. (The report was not published, but leaked to the Press: *Observer*, 11 August 1996, 21 January 1996.)

There are strong links, too, between poor health and poor housing or homelessness. Damp, unsafe homes cause illness and accidents; bed-and-breakfast accommodation is notoriously unhealthy, with high rates of infectious diseases and accidents. There are increasing numbers of water meters and self-disconnections, which the BMA and environmental health officers condemn as posing serious health risks. Homeless and badly housed women are more likely to attend ante-natal clinics late in pregnancy, to have miscarriages, to give birth prematurely, and to have babies which have low birth weights or congenital abnormalities, or die (Jones 1994).

The nature of consumer society in late twentieth-century Britain is contributing to the health risks of young people. A study of Manchester children aged between 11 and 12 found that those who were most aware of cigarette advertising were the ones most likely to take up smoking; cigarette advertising increased children's awareness of brands and encouraged them to smoke. Designer ciders and alcoholic fruit juices are the drinks most widely used by school children to get drunk, and, according to a Dundee study, growth in these brands is likely to fuel under-age drinking (*Guardian*, 16 August 1996).

A 1995 OPCS report found that children's behaviour, unemployment and homelessness are all having a serious effect on general well-being, with high levels of tobacco, alcohol, drug and volatile-substance abuse, early sexual activity, poor diets, a fall-off in physical activity and more obesity. The Government's *Health of the Nation* targets are not being met for obesity, teenage smoking or drinking among girls, and in fact the trends are in the opposite direction. Smoking among children aged between 11 and 15, for instance, has risen from 8 per cent in 1988 to 12 per cent in 1994.

(The target was 6 per cent by 1994.) Despite calls from the BMA and other groups to ban tobacco advertising, the Conservatives refused to budge (National Audit Office 1996). Moderate or severe behavioural problems were found in 7 per cent of inner-city 3-year-olds. The OPCS report concluded that class was still a major determining factor in children's health, with the exception of childhood leukaemia, which is associated with high social status (quoted in the *Guardian*, 22 September 1995). It looks as if *Health of the Nation* targets for accidents will only be met among children whose parents are in non-manual occupations. Child accident rates have fallen dramatically among the better off, but have barely moved among the poorest families, hence the class divide is widening, so that children in class 5 are five times more likely to die in accidents than children in class 1. The risk of fire is much greater in low-standard homes and in bed-and-breakfast accommodation. Children in cheap cars without modern safety devices are more likely to be killed in road accidents.

In older children the link between health and class is less pronounced than for other age groups, but it does not disappear. In families where a parent is unemployed there are material problems and stress for all the family (Department of Health 1994). There is some evidence that in the 1990s high-risk activities, such as drug abuse and abuse of solvents (such as aerosols, fuel gases and correction material), are more prevalent among poorer families. Volatile-substance abuse seems to be more common in lower socio-economic groups and where there is personal disadvantage and family problems (Home Office 1995: 1–45). There are also links among heterosexuals, including children, between material disadvantage and HIV/AIDS (Honigsbaum 1991: 18–42; Barnardos 1995: 11). In families where a member has HIV/AIDS, employment, appropriate housing and adequate income are often absent.

The threat of contracting HIV/AIDS is especially acute among children and young people engaged in prostitution. Even if they do not contract AIDS, the consequences for their health are severe, and many may already be suffering from poor health before they begin sex work. It has been estimated that as many as 5,000 children may be engaged in prostitution in Britain. A Children's Society report into child prostitution found that disruption and discord in early life, sexual abuse, neglect, school problems, unemployment and running away were all associated with children entering prostitution. Children who had been in care, moreover, were especially vulnerable to prostitution as a means of earning money, yet poverty was often a contributory factor in children being taken into care in the first place. The residential care system itself is under-resourced, with large homes run by too few staff, poorly paid and inadequately trained. Many children leaving residential homes end up on the streets, homeless and poor and with no emotional or any other kind of support. They are in no position to take up and hold down a government training place. Yet they have had no other legitimate source of income since the 1988 Social Security Act removed 16- and 17-year-olds' right to benefit except in very particular circumstances. The Children's Society has called for special training and access to benefits for homeless young people and income for children living in poverty in order to provide them with 'exit routes' from prostitution (Children's Society 1995).

The Children's Society report has since been followed by a Barnardos report on child prostitution in Bradford which unearthed evidence of children as young as 12 being imprisoned, physically and mentally tortured, and forced into prostitution. More than half had been raped by their pimps. The Barnardos report called for a Parliamentary working party on child prostitution, the decriminalisation of the abused children and a process of educating abusers (*Guardian*, 21 August 1996).

Various groups working with children and young people who are, or have been, involved in prostitution, including the Children's Society, are calling for the decriminalisation of child prostitution. In contrast, the Association of Directors of Social Services doubts that decriminalisation would have the desired effect, arguing that it may encourage pimps and others to lead more children into prostitution. What is clear is that the pimps and men who are engaged in this child abuse should be prosecuted. When men hand over money in order to abuse a child, or when men facilitate the abuse of children, it does not alter the fact that such men are child-abusers, and they should be punished accordingly. The press has highlighted the income differentials between first-world sex tourists who travel abroad to abuse children and the children they abuse; the resource inequalities between those men who pay to abuse children in their own country and the children they abuse should not be overlooked.

What, then, has been the response of governments to class-related ill health and lack of well-being among children and young people? Conservative policies and arguments between the political parties have focused on the delivery of health care: the mixed economy of health care – internal markets and general practitioner fund-holding – and rationing (or setting priorities, as politicians like to call it) are the focus of political debate, not the socio-economic influences on people's health. Yet, health care systems will have only a marginal effect on individual's lives; they are not the prime, or most direct, influence on standards of health. Attempts to change specific patterns of disease have been undertaken through the Conservatives' strategy of setting targets for reducing ill-health in five broad areas – coronary heart disease and stroke, cancer, mental illness, HIV/AIDS and sexual illnesses, and accidents – set out in a 1992 White Paper, *Health of the Nation* (Department of Health 1992). The strategy adopted has focused largely on behavioural changes, yet it has long been known that those who respond best to health education programmes are those who are already among the healthiest in society. Such a strategy can, therefore, increase inequalities between groups. As discussed above, many *Health of the Nation* targets for poorer young people are unlikely to be met.

The relationship between cultural or behavioural and material influences on standards of health are highly complex. Clare Blackburn has convincingly argued that the poor are not ignorant about healthy lifestyles, nor are their goals for their children's health lower than those of the better-off, but the socio-economic environment negatively affects the way poorer parents are able to care for, and promote the health of, their children. Further, poor parents are constantly having to set health priorities; one healthy activity may be sacrificed for another one (Blackburn 1991).

While behaviour is difficult for governments to alter, the social structure and the workings of the economy are amenable to government intervention. Governments need to pay greater attention to the likely impact of their health policies on social inequalities in standards of health, as well as to the impact on health of economic and social policies which increase material inequalities. Richard Wilkinson has argued that health in affluent societies is now less influenced by people's absolute standard of living than by their standard of living relative to others in the same society. The psycho-social factors associated with relative deprivation have a negative effect on people's health and well-being. The implications of his argument are that only by reducing inequalities and creating a less hierarchical society will standards of health continue to rise overall. Rising standards of living for some, with no redistribution of resources, will not improve aggregate figures for standards of health, let alone the health of the poorest sections of society (Wilkinson 1994). Moving towards a classless society is, therefore, relevant for future overall standards of health and health-care costs.

It is clear that wealthier families on the whole enjoy better health than poorer ones; reducing child poverty is, therefore, the most obvious route to improving the health of poorer children. The Conservatives' key policy for lone parents and their children, among the poorest families in the country, has been the Child Support Act, yet this has not produced any direct financial benefits for lone parents and their children. Most suggestions for improving the position of poor families have focused on a more generous social security system, and on changing the way it works, so that more families can escape the poverty trap of being worse off in work than on benefits. The social security budget has already become far too bloated over the last twenty years, and any further increases are not politically viable. The key to improving the life chances of children in poor families is to strengthen their parents' position in the labour market. Over the last decade the proportion of working mothers with children under the age of 5 has risen considerably, although the proportion of single mothers in paid work has fallen. A comprehensive nursery education system would give single women, in particular, greater opportunity to move into paid work and off benefits. So, from the point of view of the social security budget, investing in nursery education makes economic sense.

A comprehensive system of high quality nursery school education would facilitate the taking up of paid work of mothers, in particular those mothers bringing up children on their own, and so provide material and educational benefits for the children, and benefits to the mothers. Many women, of course, work in part-time, unskilled jobs; more time for them to undertake vocational training might improve their job and promotion prospects. The importance of a woman's place in the labour market cannot be overestimated. If women have secure work with decent wages, it helps to give them independence from undesirable men and from welfare benefits; in the long-term, it enables women to claim full National Insurance and pension entitlements. The following section sets out the case for nursery education, and goes into some detail about the specific advantages of nursery schools for children. Many politicians are eager to claim that they support nursery education in principle, but the inadequacies of their parties' policies suggest that they do not really understand what it is about nursery education that is so important, and it is rare to see the nature of high quality nursery education and its advantages detailed, except in specialist publications. Without understanding the detail, the overall advantages and case for high quality nursery education can easily be lost.

THE RIGHT START

Since the early part of the century, when educationalists emphasised the importance of nursery education, it has formed a key demand for those concerned with the inter-related health, care and educational needs of young children. Margaret McMillan, the most influential campaigner for nursery schools within Britain, who opened her own nursery school and developed training for nursery teachers, emphasised the special importance of nursery education for poor and deprived children. Nursery schools have long been recognised as having an immediate beneficial effect on children and on the wider society. McMillan argued that children should be part of the natural environment in order to improve their slum environment. Nursery schools should be surrounded by gardens, for 'The garden is the essential matter. Not the lessons, or the pictures, or the talk. . . . In the garden the child's senses and spirit are woken' (McMillan 1930: 1, 2). Playing, and playing in a garden, was all important. Partly because of the emphasis she placed on the importance of play, McMillan opposed nursery classes tacked onto infant classes. She believed that play should take place in an environment where the child was surrounded by nature, and where she could learn the importance of cleanliness, and thus develop health-enhancing life skills. All three – play, cleanliness and good health – could be promoted by baths for children at the nursery school. As a result of the environment in which slum children lived, McMillan advocated a long nursery school day of nine hours. She underlined that this did not reduce the responsibility of the mothers, but gave them new power and knowledge. This impact on the mothers was vital for McMillan, who wanted the influence of the nursery school to extend into the local community. Mothers were encouraged, therefore, to become an integral part of the school; token gestures of inviting them in for the odd show days and fêtes were simply not good enough. McMillan practised what she preached; at her nursery school in Deptford there was a weekly club for the mothers (McMillan 1930). While the tone of her writings strikes the modern-day reader as somewhat dated, the case for the type of nursery schools advocated by McMillan, and other educationalists earlier in the century, is no less relevant today.

In recent years a series of highly-respected reports and studies, including ones under governmental auspices, such as the 1990 Rumbold Report, have underlined the importance of nursery educa- tion (for more details of these, see Smith 1994). The Paul Hamlyn Foundation's National Commission on Education Report called for high-quality, publicly-funded nursery education for all 3- and 4-year- olds (National Commission on Education 1993). Co-ordination, equality of access and adequate resourcing are all common themes of those concerned with meeting the needs of young children (Pugh 1992: 9). Calls have been made for adequate pre-school education in order to improve the quality of life for young children and their parents. Its beneficial effects on cognitive development, in particular, as well as educational achievement and children's behaviour have been convincingly demonstrated (Osborn and Milbank 1987). Recently it has been claimed that high-quality early-childhood services which are comprehensive, integrated and cohesive would make for a healthy and prosperous society through their contribution to children, parents, employers and the local community (Moss and Penn 1996). On the Right, advocates of nursery education have claimed that it has benefi- cial effects on crime and unemployment rates, and other manifestations of 'not getting on well in life' (Soskin 1995).

Nursery education is particularly important to the lives of young children in today's world. Living accommodation is often confined; there is no garden or safe place for the child to play out of doors; there are no other children to play with; and home circumstances are stressful, due to poverty, unemployment, the breakdown of marriage or a partner's lack of support. Parents can be isolated as well as children, and nursery schools are a place where parents can be brought together, where they can be provided with information and where health-promotion activities can take place, in the knowl- edge that children are not falling through the net.

There is evidence that the longer a child spends in a nursery school, the greater the impact on her later school performance. Educationalists argue that nursery education is of particular advan- tage to poor and deprived children because it frees their mothers to go to work and improves their chances of performing well at primary school. The most recent research suggests that a disadvan- taged child who has attended nursery school enters the primary school with a better aptitude for education. The child impresses the teachers, who develop more positive expectations of her, and the child then directs her efforts to trying to conform to the high expectations. It is possible, too, that the positive image the teacher has of the ex-nursery school child will influence parents and their expectations of the child, and the child responds to positive labelling both at home and at school. Savings in the education budget in the long term are, therefore, also possible: special needs can be identified and remedied earlier, and drop-out rates reduced. Recent evidence from Wandsworth Council, which tests all 5-year-olds, shows that nursery education has a significantly positive effect, which is most pronounced for children on free school meals, that is, the poorest children (*Guardian*, 17 September 1996).

If children from poor and deprived backgrounds are to benefit in the short-term and the long-term, they require high-quality nursery education which is designed with their needs in mind. For this to happen, all children whose parents desire it should have access to a place in a high-quality nursery school. This demand begs the questions of what 'high quality' is, and why a nursery school is preferable to any of the other types of provision for the under-5s. The following account presents a picture of best practice in nursery schools; unless the resources are forthcoming the ideal cannot be implemented nationally.

High-quality nursery education provides a safe, caring environment where children feel wanted and valued, and where they are treated as growing individuals. Two years of nursery education for 3- to 5-year-olds gives children time to grow and develop in a world tailored to children's needs. Staff members are trained teachers who have specialised in nursery education during their training or are qualified nursery nurses – NNEBs. They accept the children and the parents as they are, culturally, linguistically and developmentally. They design opportunities for children to know themselves, to develop rounded personalities, to become aware of their potential and to gain skills appropriate to their stage of development. Nursery education is concerned with the overall development of a child, and therefore has positive implications for her health and general well-being; it is in the first few years of life that a child acquires the basic interpersonal, social, motor and mental skills needed for happy interaction with others, and as a basis for later learning.

The provision of adequate space and resources is very important, particularly if these cannot be provided at home. Young children need space indoors and outdoors in which they can move around easily and play with small and large toys and equipment. A suitable garden area is essential. The furniture, tables and chairs are all of appropriate size, and the decor and furnishings will be light and bright. The daily programme gives children opportunities for developing through educational play. Activities will be planned which encourage children to develop emotionally, socially, mentally and physically. The play world is one in which the children are in control; they organise each other, make decisions and control the situation. The member of staff will make the play educative by being involved. Through play, children are trained in positive attitudes towards learning, how to concentrate and how to apply themselves. They learn how to give and take, wait turns and consider others. In the normal way a child may not be able to concentrate for long periods, but in the play situation it will concentrate for longer periods. Failure is critical in learning, but in a play situation it does not matter to children if they 'fail'. In a nursery school time is allowed for the development of play. The quality of the play will be the sole preoccupation in the nursery teacher's mind, and the teacher is not distracted by having to rush to the shops, do the cooking or household work, or by other adults or children. Children's vocabulary can be extended through shared experience and mutual discussion. Nursery education can be especially beneficial to those ethnic-minority children living in a family which does not speak English, or only speaks it as a second language. Language and mathematical concepts will be developed through educational play for all the children. A child can enter fully into a 'child's world' at nursery school and for many this has a therapeutic benefit. Not only is a harmonious, orderly learning environment closely connected with all-round development, young children also enjoy a routine and like to know what is going to happen next.

A nursery school can provide a range of equipment which the child is highly unlikely to encounter elsewhere; the poorer the home the child comes from the less likely that the space or the money will be available for the wide range of equipment available in a nursery school. The following list, which is far from comprehensive, gives an indication of the resources of a nursery school: a fully equipped 'home corner'; dressing-up clothes; sand and water tanks with objects which sink or float; growing plants and flowers; dough, paint and crayons; musical instruments; weighing scales, paper, pencils and picture-books. In comfortable corners or rooms children can enjoy looking at picture books, listening to stories, learning nursery rhymes and jingles, finger plays, and so on. Children can spend time choosing between the various activities, which encourages motivation and the development of concentration. It does not take much imagination to realise that this range of activities and equipment is not possible in most homes, let alone poor ones, and certainly not in bed-and-breakfast accommodation. Nursery school children will not spend their days stuck in front of a television or playing in unsafe areas.

Much of the teacher/NNEB's time is spent in observing, planning, providing, teaching and recording. The nursery staff, through their observation of children, pick up clues as to what the children are capable of doing, and they can note any physical, emotional, social or learning problems; these can be referred at an early stage to the appropriate specialist. Children attending nursery schools are less isolated than those who are at home all day with one or two parents, and the problems which staff may pick up in a nursery school go well beyond purely educational ones, to those of general health and well-being; there is, for instance, more of a chance that the abuse of children will come to light, and the very fact that a child is mixing with other children and adults may operate as a constraint on an abuser. Parents can go to the nursery school to discuss their children, and to discuss the ways in which they can best help their children to learn. It is better that this advice comes from educationalists in nursery schools than from health visitors in the home, as recently suggested; offering advice with no back-up resources for parents is fraught with difficulties and echoes early-twentieth-century attempts to teach working-class mothers how to be 'better' mothers at infant welfare clinics with no financial support for them. Focusing on parenting skills should not detract from socio-economic factors which make parenting more difficult.

Gradually, children in nursery schools develop an awareness of others and their needs; they begin to appreciate nature, they are able to make simple choices, and they form stable relationships with their peers and the nursery staff. They are able to become aware of a consistent set of rules and standards of behaviour which apply to both child and adult. At the end of their time in nursery school the children are more independent and confident and are ready for the next stage of schooling.

For all the above reasons nursery school is the ideal start in life for young children. For a small minority of children a child-minder might be more appropriate than a nursery school, but for most children the experience is not sufficiently stimulating. A child-minder will lack almost all the advantages of a nursery school. A child-minder has not received the professional training of a nursery teacher or a NNEB and will not have the resources or the space of a nursery school. A home lacks diversity of equipment, and the child-minder cannot provide the breadth of experience necessary for the all-round development of the young child. Children looked after solely by a child-minder will miss out on educational play and interaction with other children of the same age; if children are left alone with a child-minder there is also scope for abuse.

Many 4-year-olds are placed in reception classes of an infant or primary school, but this again is unsuitable. In a reception class the children are part of a school which is not organised around the needs of the under-5s, so that they are constantly having to fit in with activities and an organisation designed with older children in mind. The whole ambience of infant and primary schools is different from a nursery school. Often the play times of the reception class coincides with that of older children; space in the hall is not always available for under-5s, because it is being used by older children, and the children attend assemblies, concerts and other school festivals which are not designed with under-5s' needs in mind and are not necessarily appropriate to their needs. The Head Teacher of an infant or primary school is rarely nursery trained and is, therefore, less likely to appreciate the needs of the under-5s than the Head of a nursery school. Head Teachers are keen to have as many children on the school roll as possible because money follows children, but this may not be in the best interest of the young child. There may not be adequate space for, or provision of, suitable toys and equipment in a traditional classroom, and movement within the classroom will be limited. Often there are simply not the facilities for indoor/outdoor play; few schools will have garden areas. The staff are not specially trained nursery teachers and they do not always have trained nursery assistants.

PARTY POLICY

The 1989 Children Act demonstrated a concern with the rights of children. Numerous well-received reports, including some emanating from Government, have advocated nursery school provision.

Women's need to participate in the labour market, too, has pointed to the need for nursery education, but despite both Conservatives and Labour claiming a commitment to nursery education, the reality has been very different. The provision of nursery schools in Britain lags well behind that in some of our European neighbours, in particular France and Belgium. In 1993 only 51 per cent of children under 5 attended state-maintained nursery schools or nursery classes in primary schools. In 1994, 77 per cent of 4-year-olds in England were attending Local Authority or grant-maintained schools full-time or part-time for at least part of the year before compulsory school age; 26 per cent were in nursery schools or classes, 51 per cent in primary school reception classes. The provision for the 4 million children under the age of 5 is very varied. There are Local Authority and private nursery schools, nursery classes in primary schools, and some primary schools offering full-time care to children considered by social services to be at risk; there are primary classes in which some pre-school age children are enrolled; day nurseries under social services; joint LEA and social-service nursery centres; play groups and toddlers' groups run by families or community groups; workplace crèches and child-minders. Altogether this covers roughly 90 per cent of all 3- and 4-year-olds (Department for Education and Employment 1996a; European Commission 1995).

Pressure on resources and a strategy of promoting a mixed economy of welfare, with the emphasis on choice and variety of provision, has meant that a clearly demonstrated need has not been met. The Conservative Party's scheme for meeting a pledge to provide nursery education for all 4-year-olds (and, at some time in the future, for 3-year-olds as well) was to offer nursery education vouchers worth up to £1,100 a year. In April 1996 the scheme was piloted in Norfolk and the London boroughs of Wandsworth, Westminster, and Kensington and Chelsea; there was an average 80 per cent take-up, ranging from 92 per cent in Norfolk to 55 per cent in Kensington and Chelsea. In April 1997 the scheme went nation-wide. The voucher can be used in all schools, play groups and nurseries which are part of the scheme.

The Conservatives expect the voucher to cover a part-time place, or a full-time place *if it is on offer*, in state nursery and primary schools; some Local Authority day nurseries may also join the scheme. It is likely that many of the places for older 4-year-olds will be in primary school reception classes. The voucher will cover fees up to £1,100 a year in private nursery schools and nurseries and in play groups, which should cover the costs of a daily part-time place of around two-and-a-half hours a day for at least 33 weeks a year, not including holidays. State schools will not charge any fees, but if the fees in private establishments are more than £1,100, parents will have to pay the difference; Local Authority day nurseries may also charge top-up fees. The scheme is really for parents who wish their child to attend on a part-time basis; it neither addresses the requirements of a lone parent who needs and wishes to enter the labour market, nor does it, of itself, create more places. The Conservatives assume that the money from the vouchers will encourage schools, play groups and nurseries to create more places, although a document leaked to the *Sunday Telegraph* suggests that within the Department for Education and Employment it is doubted whether this will in fact happen (*Sunday Telegraph*, 18 August 1996). It will be left to the market to provide the places; if the market does not provide them, there is no guarantee that the Government will make provision, and there is no money set aside for the capital start-up costs of new nursery schools. The scheme does not, moreover, provide nursery education dedicated to the needs of a 4-year-old; as the Conservative Government itself admitted, most of the places for older 4-year-olds will be in primary reception classes, which, as discussed above, are there to cater for an older age group with different needs. There does not appear to be money for training extra teachers and NNEBs.

The Department for Education and Employment claims that all those schools, play groups and nurseries taking part must publish information on their staff (including their qualifications) and on their premises and equipment; they must work towards a set of goals for children's learning, and they must be inspected during their first year after joining the scheme, to make sure that they are meeting the standards set (Department for Education and Employment 1996b). It is quite possible, however, that nursery schools may not be inspected for a year, which is a long time in a young child's life. Where the extra resources for this inspection (which has been sub-contracted to Group 4 to oversee) will come from is not clear, if indeed there will be extra resources. It is possible for private nurseries to get around the law which sets out staffing levels, space and inspections by taking in at least five school-age children and registering as a school (*Guardian*, 26 September 1996).

Within six months of the pilot scheme's launch, Conservative-controlled Westminster Council found it a nightmare. It doubted whether the scheme would widen choice and improve the quality of nursery education; the £1,100 was not covering the cost of even a part-time nursery place, and it was feared that the number of places might even fall (*Guardian*, 19 September 1996). In the Autumn of 1996 three of the Directors of Education in whose areas the pilot schemes operated admitted that parents were disgruntled with, and Head Teachers hostile to, the voucher system. In contrast, Ed Lister, Leader of Wandsworth Council, seemed well-satisfied with the pilot scheme in his borough. An interim report of an evaluation by the National Children's Bureau found that the scheme was having the effect of pushing 4-year-olds into starting primary school early, and concern was expressed over the quality of education these 4-year-olds were receiving. It found that, in order to meet government guidelines for learning outcomes, additional training was required for staff, but this was not happening; it also confirmed that vouchers were not covering the costs of setting up or expanding nursery schools, and the administration of the vouchers was time-consuming. Teachers in Wandsworth have called for the scheme to be abandoned. Robert Squire, minister responsible for schools, ploughed on regardless, claiming that the scheme was a 'success' (*Times Educational Supplement*, 1 November 1996; *Sunday Times*, 10 November 1996).

At the 1996 Labour Party Conference Tony Blair put education at the top of his list of priorities and claimed that he was in favour of 'proper' nursery education and opposed to vouchers. The Labour Party was already pledged to expand nursery provision, promising that within eighteen months of taking office it would guarantee every 4-year-old (later 3-year-olds as well) a year in a nursery school or play group. Again, this was not a commitment to nursery *schools*, or to full-time places. Under the Labour government, Local Authorities will be required to draw up nursery development plans in partnership with private and voluntary providers to eliminate shortages of places. The service will be free, but those choosing more expensive places outside the Local Authority sector will have to pay top-up fees (*Guardian*, 19 April 1996). The Labour Party claims that it will seek to ensure that specific support for nursery education is ring-fenced (Labour Party n.d.); it also claims that it will end the voucher system. David Blunkett has floated the idea of a pilot scheme of 25 'excellence centres', where parents can buy child care and take their 3- and 4-year-olds for nursery education, although only on a part-time basis. The idea for this suggestion comes from a scheme in North Tyneside which provides both child care and nursery education from 7.30 a.m. to 6 p.m. and is open all year. Hopefully this will provide a model, not simply an ideal to be watered down by pressure from the Treasury.

A voucher scheme means that money is spent on administering the scheme which could go direct to the schools. It is based on the premise that choice and variety is all-important, yet research has underlined the importance of nursery schools of high quality, with specific curricula, and it is these that need to be made available nation-wide, rather than a range of provision that varies in quality, and some of which has little proven benefit to children. Both parties are pledged to extend nursery provision to 3-year-olds, but the timing and funding are still vague. Neither party has taken on board either the specific advantages of nursery schools over other forms of pre-school provision or of offering genuine full-time places for those children whose parents want them.

The Liberal Democrats appear to have the best-thought-out proposals. They criticise the existing patchy provision on the grounds that variable nursery education means unequal opportunities right from the start. They claim that they would provide nursery education for all 3- and 4-year-olds, within the lifetime of a Parliament. They emphasise the need for high-quality nursery education, for appropriate training for the extra teachers and NNEBs required, and in-service training for those already working in nursery education. The Liberal Democrats have pledged to devote an extra penny in the pound of income tax to education, and to prioritise nursery education. They have estimated that capital costs will be roughly £1.5 billion over five years, which includes training 18,000 new teachers and 2,000 ancillary staff, but the creation of 44,000 new jobs would create savings (if all the new staff were recruited from among the unemployed the saving in benefits would be in the region of £370 million). They estimate annual revenue costs to be £860 million (Liberal Democrats n.d.). On paper, the Liberal Democrats' policy looks the best, but, while they can influence the climate of opinion in which Government policy is drawn up and have a direct influence at the local level, the Liberal Democrats will not be determining national policy.

CONCLUSION

Those who reap the greatest benefits from the education system are, on the whole, the most privileged sections of society. Not so with nursery education: it offers greatest benefits to the least privileged in our society. If we want to create a more classless and less racialised society, a comprehensive nursery education system is a good place to start. Nursery education can help to reduce a family's poverty and give a child a good start in the education system. It therefore contributes to the health and well-being of children and adults, for, as we have seen, standards of health are still closely related to class position. Of course, it is not a panacea for all the ills associated with poverty – solvent abuse and child prostitution will not disappear once all children have had a nursery school education – but it is a means of tackling the problems associated with poverty early on in a child's life and of addressing health problems from a wide perspective. Nursery education for all 3- to 5-year-olds is not an unrealistic, utopian idea; it is within the realms of political possibility, and it offers a strategy for moving towards a classless society. It is, moreover, not an alarming policy for those politicians uninterested in, or hostile to, the idea of a less class-ridden society: for them the merits of nursery education can be seen in the way that it inculcates desirable behaviour in children and creates the circumstances in which single mothers can seek paid work, so contributing to a breakdown in the alleged 'dependency culture'.

REFERENCES

Barker, D. *et al.* (1989) 'Weight in infancy and death from ischaemic heart disease', *Lancet* ii: 577–80.

Barnardos (1995) *No Time to Waste: The Scale and Dimensions of the Problem of Children Affected by HIV/AIDS in the United Kingdom*, London: Barnardos.

Blackburn, C. (1991) *Poverty and Health: Working With Families*, Milton Keynes: Open University Press.

Bundey, S., Alam, H., Kaur, A., Mir, S. and Lancashire, R. (1991) 'Why do UK-born Pakistani babies have high perinatal and neonatal mortality rates?', *Paediatric and Perinatal Epidemiology*, January: 101–14.

Children's Society (1995) *The Game's Up: Redefining Child Prostitution*, London: Children's Society.

Department for Education and Employment (1996a) *Nursery Education Scheme: The Next Steps*, London: Department for Education and Employment.

—— (1996b) *Nursery Education Vouchers: A Guide for Parents*, London: Department for Education and Employment.

Department of Health (1990) *On the State of the Public Health*, London: HMSO.

—— (1992) *The Health of the Nation: A Strategy for Health in England*, London: HMSO.

—— (1994) *On the State of the Public Health*, London: HMSO.

European Commission (1995) *Pre-school Education in the EU: Current Thinking and Practice*, Education Training Youth Studies, No. 6. Luxembourg: Office for Official Publications of the European Communities.

Home Office (1995) *Advisory Council on the Misuse of Drugs: Volatile Substance Abuse*, London: HMSO.

Honigsbaum, N. (1991) *HIV, AIDS and Children: A Cause for Concern*, London: National Children's Bureau.

Jones, H. (1994) *Health and Society in Twentieth-Century Britain*, London: Longman.

Labour Party (n.d.) *The Best Start*, London: Labour Party.

Liberal Democrats (n.d.) *Making the Right Start: A Liberal Democrat Consultation Paper on Nursery Education and Care*, London: Liberal Democrat Party.

McMillan, M. (1930) *The Nursery School*, London: Dent. (First published 1919).

Moss, P. and Penn, H. (1996) *Transforming Nursery Education*, London: Paul Chapman.

National Audit Office (1996) *Health of the Nation: A Progress Report*, London: HMSO.

National Commission on Education (1993) *Learning to Succeed: A Radical Look at Education Today and a Strategy for the Future*, London: Heinemann.

Osborn, A.F. and Milbank, J.E. (1987) *The Effects of Early Education: A Report from the Child Health and Education Study*, Oxford: Clarendon Press.

Power, C. *et al.* (1990) 'Health in childhood and social inequalities in health in young adults', *Journal of the Royal Statistical Society* 153(1): 17–28.

Pugh, G. (1992) 'A policy for early childhood services?', in G. Pugh (ed.) *Contemporary Issues in the Early Years: Working Collaboratively for Children*, London: Paul Chapman.

Smith, E. (1994) *Educating the Under-5s*, London: Cassell.

Soskin, D. (1995) *Pre-Schools For All: A Market Solution*, London: Adam Smith Institute.

Townsend, P. and Davidson, N. (1982) *Inequalities in Health: The Black Report*, Harmondsworth: Penguin.

Wilkinson, R. (1994) 'Health, redistribution and growth', in A. Glyn and D. Miliband (eds) *Paying for Inequality: The Economic Cost of Social Injustice*, London: IPPR/Rivers Oram Press.

Chapter 4

Education and the reproduction of class-based inequalities

Andy Furlong

INTRODUCTION

Recent changes in young people's educational experiences have important implications for labour-market transitions and pose some fundamental questions for our understanding of processes of social reproduction in advanced industrial societies. In Britain, the restructuring of the youth labour market during the 1980s had a particularly significant impact on patterns of educational participation (Ashton et al. 1990). With the decline of manufacturing industry, the virtual collapse of the youth labour market and the subsequent restructuring of employment opportunities for young workers, employers were able to demand more advanced educational qualifications and different types of skills, which, in turn, meant that the average age at which young people entered the labour market increased (Ashton et al. 1990; Furlong 1992; Roberts 1995; Furlong and Cartmel 1997). Moreover, with unemployment and training schemes becoming central to the experiences of a growing proportion of young people, routes involving extended education started to appear more attractive (Raffe and Willms 1989). As a result of these changes, by the late 1980s young people tended to follow a wider and much more diverse set of routes through the education system and into the labour market than had been the case a decade earlier (Furlong and Cartmel 1997). For sociologists these changes are particularly significant, because within industrial societies educational experiences have long been regarded as central to the reproduction of socio-economic inequalities. Although the most prestigious positions in the labour market tend to be allocated to those with strong educational qualifications, social class has long been regarded as one of the best predictors of academic attainment (Halsey et al. 1980; Furlong 1992). With education playing such an important role in the process of social reproduction, any trend towards the establishment of a 'classless' society should be manifest in a significant weakening of the relationship between social class and educational experiences. In this context, it is important to assess the extent to which changes in patterns of schooling and the increase in certification has led to an equalisation of educational outcomes. As such, the first theme to be addressed in this chapter relates to the question of whether social class is still central to an understanding of the routes which young people follow through education and of the sorts of qualifications which they gain.

Although it is argued that social class has remained central to an understanding of educational experiences, the fact that young people remain in full-time education for significantly longer periods and follow a more diverse set of educational routes does have implications for processes of social reproduction. In particular, an increased emphasis on credentials and the greater social mix within educational institutions can be seen as having weakened collective responses to the school. Whereas educational experiences were once strongly class-differentiated, today young people spend more time in socially mixed educational environments. In this context, the second theme of this chapter explores the question of whether recent educational changes have had a significant impact on the subjective reproduction of classes within the school.

SCHOOLS AND THE REPRODUCTION OF SOCIO-ECONOMIC INEQUALITIES

In capitalist societies, the unequal distribution of social and economic rewards has often been justified in terms of the opportunities which people receive, and schools play an important role in preparing young people for the positions they will enter in the occupational hierarchy. With education being available to everyone, schools have frequently been seen as standing between family background and labour-market position and, according to functionalists, help to ensure that the most able and best-qualified people are placed in the most demanding jobs (Davis and Moore 1945). While few modern sociologists adhere to functionalist perspectives, it can be argued that if Britain is on the road to becoming a 'classless' society then we would expect to see an improvement in the position of pupils from less-advantaged backgrounds within the school.

Over the last two decades there have been important changes in the education system which have had a powerful impact on young people's experience of schooling. Following the 'Great Debate' on education initiated by James Callaghan in 1976, a number of educational changes were introduced during the 1980s, due to concerns about shortages of qualified recruits for industry and as a result of fears that education was not organised in such a way as to promote the efficient development of human resources. In the three decades following the 1944 Education Act, educational reforms were frequently motivated by concerns about social justice: in particular, there was a commitment to reducing the 'wastage' of working-class talent in an education system which traditionally favoured pupils from advantaged social backgrounds. Yet, while the educational reforms introduced in the post-war period have had an impact on the school experiences of young people from working-class families, evidence associating these changes with a process of equalisation has been deceptive.

Despite the common belief that ascribed occupational roles have gradually been eroded, the truth of the matter is that social ascent through education is limited, and family background has remained an important determinant of educational attainment throughout this century (Halsey *et al.* 1980; Gray *et al.* 1983; Shavit and Blossfeld 1993; Furlong and Cartmel 1997). Indeed, sociologists have frequently argued that in advanced capitalist societies educational systems are central to the legitimation of inequalities (Sarup 1982). Bourdieu, for example, argues that it is through education that those from less-advantaged backgrounds come to associate their failure with individual shortcoming. As a consequence of an 'ideology of giftedness', people come to 'see as natural inability things which are only the result of an inferior social status' (Bourdieu 1974: 42). Despite meritocratic principles and a façade of openness, the British educational system effectively guarantees success to a large proportion of the offspring of those occupying advantaged positions in the socio-economic order.

The close association between socio-economic position and educational performance reflects the impact of both economic and cultural resources. On an economic level, many researchers have drawn attention to the relationship between material disadvantage and school performance. During this century many of the improvements in the performance of working-class pupils have been seen as a consequence of changes in the material circumstances of families – rather than of specific educational reforms – and as affected by factors such as the post-war slum-clearance programme, a reduction in overcrowding and the development of the welfare state (Plowden Report 1967).

While the link between material deprivation and under-achievement is certainly important, sociologists have also argued that cultural resources are central to an understanding of educational disadvantage (Jackson and Marsden 1962; Willis 1977; Furlong 1993). Bernstein (1971), for example, suggested that the acquisition of different lingual codes by children from different social-class backgrounds affects the schools' view of the ability of the child. In a similar vein, Bourdieu (1973, 1974) has argued that middle-class advantages in the educational system are largely due to the similarity between middle-class culture and the dominant culture, and that the mode of learning employed in schools is similar to that practised within middle-class families: 'Teachers assume that they already share a common language and set of values with their pupils', but the lower classes 'only acquire with great effort something which is given to the children of the cultivated classes' (Bourdieu 1974: 39). Other sociologists, such as Willis (1977) and Jenkins (1983), have argued that the normative orientations of young people themselves are of prime importance in determining educational success. In this respect, the generally poor academic performance of young people from lower working-class backgrounds has been seen as a consequence of their rejection of 'success' as defined in middle-class terms. Working-class lifestyles often emphasise different sets of values and priorities from middle-class styles of life (Willis 1977; Jenkins 1983). There tends to be a conflict between academic success, which requires a postponement of immediate rewards in order to gain future advan-tages, and working-class values, which stress the importance of enjoyment in the here-and-now (Ashton and Field 1976). The view that working-class pupils do not regard educational success as important has been challenged by Brown (1987), who argues that many approach the school instrumentally and regard education as a means through which they can enhance their employment prospects. More recent evidence supports this view (Biggart and Furlong 1996), yet it is important to remember that working-class pupils are frequently disadvantaged at school, despite a desire to succeed.

EDUCATIONAL CHANGE AND THE MAINTENANCE OF CLASS-BASED DIFFERENTIALS

Recent changes in the organisation of schooling have had an important impact on the ways in which inequalities are reproduced, although many reforms have failed to live up to initial expectations. Comprehensive education, for example, was introduced as a means of providing a greater social mix within schools, which, in turn, would aid the academic performance of lower-class pupils. However, the continued use of ability streams within Comprehensive schools has been seen as reinforcing the effects of social class. Ball (1981), for example, has suggested that banding in Comprehensive schools has resulted in a system which is no fairer in terms of equality of opportunity than the selective system which it replaced. During the late 1980s and early 1990s a number of new vocational courses have been introduced, which have been seen as helping make the upper secondary school less elitist (Raffe 1992). Whereas the upper secondary school was once centred around a highly academic curriculum, the range of courses on offer to less academic pupils has become much broader, and there has been a significant increase in the number of young people remaining in education after the age of 16. In the context of these educational reforms, in this section I examine the impact of these changes on the reproduction of socio-economic inequalities.

Over the last decade, rates of participation in post-compulsory education have increased rapidly among all social groups. These changes have had a significant effect on the class-composition of the upper secondary school and are further reflected in the transformation of higher education from an elite experience to a mass phenomenon. Whereas socially differentiated educational experiences were once a key feature of the British educational system, recent changes have led to a greater commonality of experience. Prior to Comprehensivisation, the educational experiences of working-class and middle-class pupils were quite distinct: most working-class pupils were placed in Secondary Modern schools, while middle-class children frequently obtained places in Grammar schools. While the introduction of Comprehensive schools has led to a greater social mix within institutions, in practice many class-based divisions have remained intact. In particular, a strong correlation has been observed between social class and the streams to which young people were allocated (Ball 1981). Moreover, working-class pupils have tended to leave school at an earlier stage (frequently at the minimum age) and obtain fewer qualifications than their middle-class counterparts. Indeed, although there have been significant changes in the organisation of education, one of the lessons which we learn from recent history is that greater access to education is not necessarily reflected in a reduction in class-based inequalities (Shavit and Blossfeld 1993). The 1944 Education Act, for example, was introduced with the explicit aim of providing more equal access to educational opportunities, yet subsequent analysis of the impact of the reforms showed that class-based differences in educational experiences remained firmly entrenched (Halsey *et al.* 1980).

While there is some evidence that Comprehensive schools have had a positive effect on levels of attainment of working-class youth, these changes have been relatively small. Using Scottish data, McPherson and Willms (1987) argued that between 1976 and 1984 a process of 'equalisation' took place, as pupils with a socio-economic status (SES) one standard deviation below the national average increased their attainment relative to pupils of average SES. This improvement in performance was in the region of one O grade pass for males and half an O grade pass for females.[1] However, this trend did not extend to the upper levels of attainment, nor to the post-compulsory stages of secondary schooling. In other words, this improvement is unlikely to have a radical impact on patterns of social reproduction. In order to make a fuller assessment of the significance of changes in the British educational system for the reproduction of social classes, it is necessary to review the extent to which patterns of participation and educational outcomes have changed over the last few years. National statistics show that in 1984/5 less than half (48 per cent) of all 16-year-olds remained in education beyond the minimum leaving age; by 1994/5 almost three-quarters (73 per cent) remained in full-time education (Department of Education and Employment 1995). Over the same period, full-time educational participation among the 16 to 18 age group increased from less than a third (32 per cent) to nearly six in ten (57 per cent). These changing patterns of post-compulsory educational participation between 1976 and 1992 are illustrated in Figure 4.1. Aside from highlighting a sharp rise in participation between the mid-1980s and early 1990s, this chart also highlights the widening gap in the participation rates of males and females: in 1976 the participation rate of females was 2 percentage points higher than males, by 1992 it had increased to 7 percentage points.

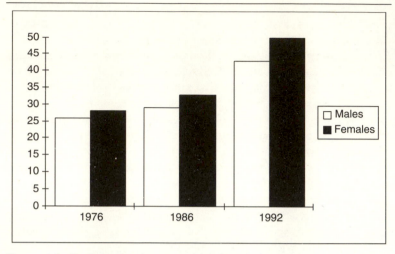

Figure 4.1   Participation in post-compulsory education –
16–18-year-olds
Source: Department for Education and Employment (1995)

While young people have become more likely to return to full-time education after the age of 16, in the context of this discussion the question which needs to be addressed relates to the persistence of class-based inequalities. Data from the England and Wales Youth Cohort Study shows quite clearly that there is still an important relationship between social class and educational participation. In 1991, post-compulsory participation ranged from almost eight in ten (78 per cent) among the professional and managerial classes, to four in ten (40 per cent) among those with parents in semi-skilled and unskilled occupations. However, comparing these figures with those from 1985 shows some evidence that the class effect on post-compulsory participation has weakened: during this period the most significant growth in participation occurred among the manual classes. While young people from the professional and managerial classes increased their participation by 8 percentage points, those from the skilled manual, and semi-skilled and unskilled manual classes increased their participation by 24 and 17 percentage points respectively (Figure 4.2). Indeed, by the early 1990s staying on at school had become a relatively common part of the post-16 experiences of young people from all social classes.

The growth in post-compulsory educational participation has been reflected in a generalised improvement in attainment levels: males and females from all social classes have become more likely to

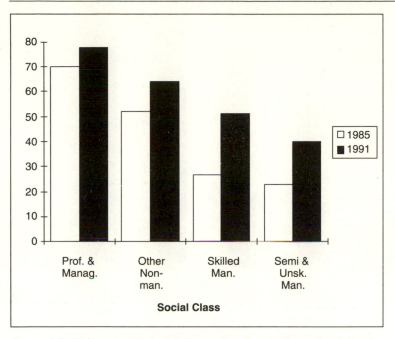

Figure 4.2   Young people in full-time education in the spring following
            the minimum school leaving age
Source: Data from the England and Wales Youth Cohort Study

obtain a graded examination result at the end of compulsory
schooling, and the chances of gaining the qualifications which
would allow them to apply for higher education have increased.
National statistics show that in 1980/1, around one in four young
people (24 per cent of males and 26 per cent of females) gained five
or more GCSEs at grades A–C. By 1993/4 almost four in ten males
(39 per cent) and nearly five in ten females (48 per cent) gained five
or more GCSEs. The proportion of young people gaining three or
more A levels also increased: from 10 per cent of males and 8 per
cent of females in 1980/1 to 14 per cent of males and 15 per cent of
females in 1993/4 (Figure 4.3).

Despite the growth in certification and the improvement in
performance, strong class differentials can still be observed, with
class-based differentials narrowing much more significantly for
females than for males. Figures for 1991 from the Scottish Young
People's Surveys show that 68 per cent of females and 60 per cent of
males from the professional and managerial classes gained five or
more O grades; the corresponding figures for the lower working

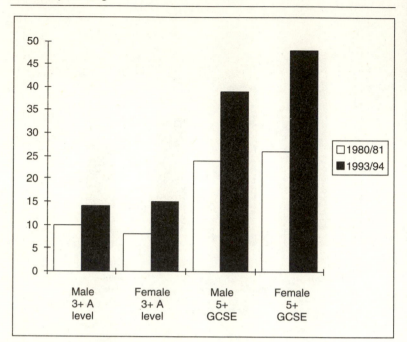

Figure 4.3   Qualifications – 1980/1 and 1993/4
Source: Central Statistical Office (1996)

classes were 25 per cent and 21 per cent for females and males respectively. In other words, while important changes in attainment can be identified, it is clear that strong class-based differentials have been maintained (Figure 4.4). On the other hand, significant changes have occurred for young women. If we look at the gains made over the period 1979 to 1991, it is clear that in each social class the rate of improvement for young women was much more pronounced than for young men. Indeed, in the late 1970s and early 1980s, gender-based differences in performance in each social class were small: by the early 1990s gender differentials had widened to such an extent that lower working-class girls were only a short distance behind upper working-class boys.

A similar pattern emerges in respect of changes in the proportion of young people who gain sufficient qualifications to apply to university. Between 1979 and 1991 the proportion of females gaining three or more Highers increased much more rapidly than that of males, yet class-based differences remained firmly entrenched (Furlong and Cartmel 1997). During this period the

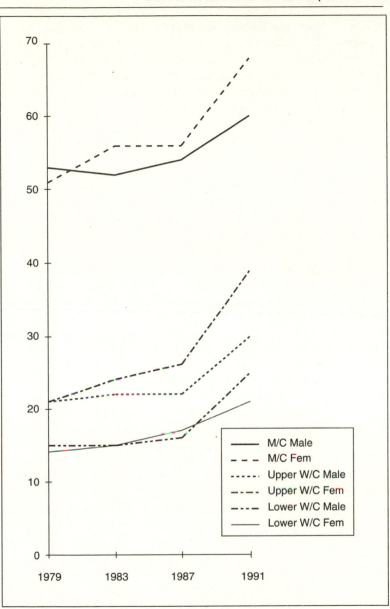

Figure 4.4   Young people gaining five or more O grades
Source: Data from the Scottish Young People's Surveys

greatest gains were made by middle-class females (up by 22 percentage points), followed by females from the upper working classes (up by 19 percentage points). Middle-class males and lower working-class females increased their chances of obtaining three or more Highers by a similar amount (14 percentage points), while the slowest rates of increase were found among upper and lower working-class boys (up by 11 and 9 percentage points respectively). With an increasing number of young people participating in full-time, post-compulsory education, and with an expansion in university places in the early 1990s, there has also been a significant growth in higher education. Between 1984/5 and 1994/5 the number of students enrolling for full-time undergraduate courses more than doubled. During this period, the number of female undergraduates rose particularly rapidly: whereas in 1984/5 40 per cent of first year undergraduates were female, by 1994/95 this had increased to 49 per cent (Department of Education and Employment 1995).

During the 1960s higher education was the preserve of a small, and largely middle-class, academic elite, but by the 1990s it had become less socially exclusive. With more than six in ten young people being likely to enrol on a course of higher education at some stage in their lives (Smithers and Robinson 1995), the chances of a young person from a working-class family obtaining a degree has certainly increased in absolute terms. However, in relative terms it can be argued that the middle classes have retained many of their previous advantages (Blackburn and Jarman 1993). After comparing four representative sample surveys conducted in 1949, 1972, 1983 and 1987, Heath and Clifford (1990) argued that, despite significant changes in the educational expectations of the population, there was little evidence of a narrowing of relative class inequalities in access to higher education.

Although it is possible to identify some far-reaching changes in the British educational system, it is clear that the advantages of those from middle-class families have largely been preserved. Working-class youth may remain in full-time education for longer periods of time, and may spend more time in socially mixed educational environments, but attainments are still strongly differentiated by class. In this respect, it is difficult to argue that any real moves towards 'classlessness' are apparent. However, there have been some significant changes in the relative performance of boys and girls which suggest that for young women the relationship between class and attainment is becoming weaker. These changes are likely to be linked to the development of the service sector and the growth of female labour-market participation, which have been reflected in modified patterns of gender socialisation. Paid work has become much more central to the lives of women, and girls are perhaps more inclined to strive for higher-level jobs which increasingly carry positive images of femininity.

SUBJECTIVE DIMENSIONS OF SOCIAL REPRODUCTION

Although the relationship between social class and educational performance has remained strong, there have been significant changes in young people's experiences within the school. In particular, an increased demand for credentials can be seen as having weakened collective approaches to schooling, while the growth of the upper secondary school and higher education has reduced the social exclusivity of educational routes. Potentially, these changes have implications for processes of social reproduction on a subjective level. With a decline in manual employment and changing labour-market experiences among working-class families, young people in the 1990s tend to develop responses towards education and the labour market that are different from those held by members of earlier generations (Biggart and Furlong 1996; Furlong and Cartmel 1997). As contexts have changed, young people have adapted the cultural responses of the previous generation to forms which are more compatible with labour demand in a modern, post-industrial economy. In this context, changes in the labour market and qualification inflation have had an important impact on the orientations of working-class youth towards the school and the job market. Whereas responses could once be described as collectivist, today they have become more individualised (Beck 1992).

In the 1960s and 1970s the process of schooling was highly differentiated, and educational experiences were strongly affected by social class. During this period sociologists frequently regarded working-class responses to the school as characterised by a cultural 'resistance': young people from working-class families frequently regarded the culture of the school as alien and developed counter-cultures in which the importance of academic success was challenged (Willis 1977; Hall and Jefferson 1976). In this respect, the educational experiences of working-class youth were collectivist: they typically left the middle-class environment of the school at the earliest opportunity in order to confirm their working-class cultural identities in the sphere of employment. In contrast, middle-class pupils tended to share the assumptive worlds and cultural values of their teachers and followed more diverse and individualised routes between school and work. These contrasting experiences of schooling meant that young people's identities were frequently developed in socially restricted networks, and they tended to develop frames of reference which reflected established class and gender relationships (Furlong and Cartmel 1997).

Today, with few job opportunities available to unqualified school-leavers, qualifications have become more significant in smoothing labour market transitions, and employers are placing a greater emphasis on personal profiles (Ashton *et al.* 1990; Banks *et al.* 1992). Especially in labour markets where there is a severe shortage of opportunities, a good reference or an extra examination pass can affect job chances. As visible resistance to the school or a lack of qualifications can increase the chances of unemployment, young people have become much more concerned about academic attainment and tend to display their opposition in more subtle ways (Biggart and Furlong 1996). Working-class youth frequently hold high educational aspirations without fully conforming to the academic ethos of the school. These contradictions are highlighted in a recent study by Biggart and Furlong (1996) as expressed here by 'Paul':

Paul [talking about Highers]: Four highers, English, Maths, Chemistry, and Physics, and I got four C's at the end. I could have done a lot better I think. I am quite sure I could have. But I ended up I wasn't too . . . in too fit a state for any of my Highers either, doing any exams, so I was quite happy to come away with four C's out of it all you know. I was smoking a lot that day [cannabis]. Some of my pals were nae taking any Highers and they thought it was dead funny that we were going in for your Highers to get you wrecked. They are like that 'going for a wee joint' and you're like that 'aye, all right'. And I ended up getting full of it and then going into the exam, wrecked sort of thing. But I could have done better than four C's but I was quite happy to get them because I knew that on the other side I could have completely ruined all my hopes you know and got nothing.

These conflicts are particularly visible in the upper secondary school, where there has been a substantial growth in 'non-traditional' stayers over the last decade (Hammer and Furlong 1996). Whereas the majority of post-compulsory school pupils used to share the social background and cultural values of their teachers, members of the new upper school are a more diverse group both culturally and academically (Biggart and Furlong 1996). Many young people from working-class families still tend to feel ill-at-ease in the academic environment of the school and are frequently torn between the conflicting pressures which arise within peer and family groups. While schools now make greater efforts to provide for pupils who fall outside the traditional academic mainstream (Raffe 1992), and while the social composition of the secondary school has changed, middle-class 'cultural capital' (Bourdieu 1973) still provides educational advantages. In this respect, social class still has an impact on school experiences.

CONCLUSION

The evidence presented in this chapter has highlighted the significant changes in young people's educational experiences which have occurred over the last two decades. Rates of participation in post-compulsory schooling have increased rapidly, and more young people are leaving full-time education with qualifications which may smooth their entry into the labour market. While these changes are important, I have suggested that traditional structures of social inequality remain intact, and that evidence to support the idea that a 'classless' society is emerging is weak. Social class is still central to an understanding of educational outcomes and the advantages of the middle classes have largely been preserved throughout a period of rapid change in education and the labour market. However, despite these central continuities, there is evidence of a weakening of class divisions among young women which is likely to be a consequence of changes in the labour market and of new forms of gender socialisation. In terms of qualifications, the greatest gains have been made by young women.

Although these continuities in objective processes of social reproduction point towards the maintenance of class society, there have been some changes in the ways young people experience schooling which suggest that subjectivities associated with class have weakened. In particular, there is evidence that responses to the school have become more individualised, and that a convergence of class-based educational experiences is helping to obscure structural continuities. In these circumstances, changes in the educational system can be seen as providing a powerful source of legitimacy in advanced capitalism, with young people increasingly regarding educational failure as a personal shortcoming rather than a consequence of their social position.

No matter which party is in power, it is difficult to imagine that significant moves will be made to weaken the links between social class and educational attainment. Many of the policies being proposed by 'New' Labour prioritise 'choice' rather than social justice and are likely to lead to the continued erosion of the socially mixed learning environments which offer some hope for the development of a more egalitarian society.

NOTE

1   An O grade can be regarded as the Scottish equivalent of a GCSE at grades A–C.

REFERENCES

Ashton, D.N. and Field, D. (1976) *Young Workers*, London: Hutchinson.

Ashton, D.N., Maguire, M.J. and Spilsbury, M. (1990) *Restructuring the Labour Market: The Implications for Youth*, Basingstoke: Macmillan.

Ball, S.J. (1981) *Beachside Comprehensive: A Case Study of Secondary Schooling*, Cambridge: Cambridge University Press.

Banks, M., Bates, I., Breakwell, G., Bynner, J., Emler, N., Jamieson, L. and Roberts, K. (1992) *Careers and Identities*, Milton Keynes: Open University Press.

Beck, U. (1992) *Risk Society: Towards a New Modernity*, London: Sage.

Bernstein, B. (1971) *Class, Codes and Control*, London: Routledge & Kegan Paul.

Biggart, A. and Furlong, A. (1996) 'Educating "discouraged workers": Cultural diversity in the upper secondary school', *British Journal of Sociology of Education* 17: 253–66.

Blackburn, R.M. and Jarman, J. (1993) 'Changing inequalities in access to British universities', *Oxford Review of Education* 19(2): 197–215.

Bourdieu, P. (1973) 'Cultural reproduction and social reproduction', in R. Brown (ed.) *Knowledge, Education and Cultural Change*, London: Tavistock.

—— (1974) 'The school as a conservative force: Scholastic and cultural inequalities', in J. Eggleston (ed.) *Contemporary Research in the Sociology of Education*, London: Methuen.

Brown, P. (1987) *Schooling Ordinary Kids*, London: Tavistock.

Central Statistical Office (1996) *Social Trends 26*, London: HMSO.

Davis, K. and Moore, W.E. (1945) 'Some principles of stratification',

American Sociological Review 18: 394–7.

Department for Education and Employment (1995) *Education Statistics for the UK*, London: HMSO.

Furlong, A. (1992) *Growing Up in a Classless Society? School to Work Transitions*, Edinburgh: Edinburgh University Press.

—— (1993) *Schooling for Jobs*, Aldershot: Avebury.

Furlong, A. and Cartmel, F. (1997) *Young People and Social Change: Individualization and Risk in Late Modernity*, Buckingham: Open University Press.

Gray, J., McPherson, A.F. and Raffe, D. (1983) *Reconstructions of Secondary Education: Theory, Myth and Practice Since the War*, London: Routledge & Kegan Paul.

Hall, S. and Jefferson, T. (1976) (eds) *Resistance Through Rituals: Youth Subcultures in Post-War Britain*, London: Hutchinson.

Halsey, A.H., Heath, A.F. and Ridge, J.M. (1980) *Origins and Destinations: Family, Class and Education in Modern Britain*, Oxford: Clarendon.

Hammer, T. and Furlong, A. (1996) 'Staying on: The effects of recent changes in educational participation for 17–19 year-olds in Norway and Scotland', *The Sociological Review* 44: 693–709.

Heath, A.F. and Clifford, P. (1990) 'Class inequalities in education in the twentieth century', *Journal of the Royal Statistical Society*, series A, 153: 1–16.

Jackson, B. and Marsden, B. (1962) *Education and the Working Class*, London: Routledge & Kegan Paul.

Jenkins, R. (1983) *Lads, Citizens and Ordinary Kids*, London: Routledge & Kegan Paul.

McPherson, A.F. and Willms, J.D. (1987) 'Equalisation and improvement: Some effects of comprehensive re-organisation in Scotland', *Sociology* 21: 509–39.

Plowden Report (1967) *Children and their Primary Schools: Report of the Central Advisory Council for Education (England), vols. I and II*, London: HMSO.

Raffe, D. (1992) 'Participation of 16–19 year-olds in education and training', *Briefing Paper No. 3*, London: National Commission on Education.

Raffe, D. and Willms, J.D. (1989) 'Schooling the discouraged worker: Local labour-market effects on educational participation', *Sociology* 23: 559–81.

Roberts, K. (1995) *Youth and Employment in Modern Britain*, Oxford: Oxford University Press.

Sarup, M. (1982) *Education, State and Crisis: A Marxist Perspective*, London: Routledge & Kegan Paul.

Shavit, Y. and Blossfeld, H.P. (1993) *Persistent Inequality*, Boulder, CO: Westview.

Smithers, A. and Robinson, P. (1995) *Post-18 Education: Growth, Change, Prospect*, London: Council for Industry and Higher Education.

Willis, P. (1977) *Learning to Labour*, Farnborough: Saxon House.

Chapter 5

Youth training

Kenneth Roberts

INTRODUCTION

By the time this chapter is read it is quite likely that Youth Training (YT) will have become history, one of the more expensive policy failures of the 1980s and 1990s. Whichever party is governing Britain is likely to have introduced a new package of measures for the twenty-first century, or so the launch will have said. We are likely to have been told that the latest package really will widen the life chances of disadvantaged young people and equip Britain with a world-class work-force. The same claims were made when the Youth Training Scheme (as it was called until 1990) began in 1983.

CLASS AND INEQUALITY

It should surprise no one that YT failed to achieve objectives that were never intended or even considered. The YTS was not supposed to make Britain a classless society in the sociological meaning of this term. It was designed to promote skills, competitiveness and enterprise – not equality or classlessness, which themselves are rather different things. There can be inequalities without class divisions, though it is impossible to envisage class divisions without inequalities.

Socio-economic equality has never been a goal of any of modern Britain's main political parties, nor a widespread aspiration. Narrowing inequalities, which is rather different, has been favoured, generally by members of less privileged groups and political parties of the Left. In contrast, it was no secret that in the 1980s the UK Government believed that inequalities needed to be widened in the interests of justice (allowing individuals to benefit from their own industry) and incentives. Economic inequalities were therefore widened deliberately and blatantly, and the presiding Government was re-elected on successive occasions. YTS, however, was not part of this particular programme.

The scheme was about opportunities. Outside sociology, classlessness is most likely to mean equal opportunities – giving equally worthy individuals the same chances to achieve the good things in life, irrespective of family background, race, sex, religion and so on. This is what most members of the public, and politicians of both Left and Right, are most likely to mean when they talk of eradicating class divisions, and it was in this sense that the YTS was supposed to assist in making Britain classless. The scheme was introduced at the time when the Prime Minister was declaring that, 'there is no such thing as society'. It was individuals who counted, and, in this view of the just world, governments and other institutions had to be dissuaded from creating or maintaining unnecessary barriers to individuals achieving their own aims.

Nowadays there is a 'tough' version of equal opportunities which equates the goal with equal outcomes. According to this view, equalising opportunities means creating the conditions wherein the ultimate achievements of members of different social groups – sex, ethnic, religious and regional groups for example – become indistinguishable. In other words, identical proportions of males and females, and black and white employees, and so on, should be in managerial jobs, and unemployed. This manner of operationalising the equal opportunities idea has been popular among pressure groups seeking better treatment for women and ethnic minorities. This 'tough' stance insists that we recognise the existence of a problem while outcomes remain unequal. Critics counter-argue that equal opportunities will only lead to equal outcomes when the groups concerned do not differ in other relevant ways, such as their values, aspirations or abilities. Whether YTS's architects hoped or intended to establish equal opportunities in the 'tough' sense was unclear. However, there were no indications that anyone believed that the scheme would make young people's future life chances independent of their past achievements in education – or, therefore, of their family backgrounds, which were known to be strongly related to success in school.

However, there is a 'soft' version of equal opportunities which enjoys wider support, including that of all Britain's main political parties, which focuses on processes rather than outcomes. It equates equalising opportunities with removing barriers which serve no one's interests – or merely sectional interests – and offering 'helping hands', thereby creating routes through which individuals with the ability and inclination can realise their ambitions. The particular barriers and helping hands (or their absence) that arouse people's passions are likely to depend on their particular social locations. People are usually most sensitive to their own, rather than other groups', situations. Some may feel it important that in recent times it has proved possible for a grocer's daughter and a circus artist's son to become prime ministers of the UK. A larger number of households are likely to have been more concerned about their members' chances of gaining any employment.

YTS was not intended to create routes into the cabinet or the business elite. Rather, the intention was to enable young people who were otherwise excluded, but who had the desire and the ability, to become qualified for skilled jobs. This was the kind of equal opportunity – classlessness some might say – that the YTS was supposed to promote. It is against this relatively modest goal, and not its failure to narrow general socio-economic inequalities or equalise the life chances of children born into privilege and poverty, that the scheme failed, and it is important that the reasons for its failure should be widely understood, if only to prevent further costly policy mistakes.

THE PROBLEM

The YTS was not a hastily conceived panic measure. It was carefully designed to address a long-standing problem. Most of the background work, which began in the 1970s, was undertaken by the Manpower Services Commission (MSC), which had been created earlier in the decade to bring a more professional approach to the management of the (then) Department of Employment's services. The MSC itself was a product of the era of consensus politics and corporatism. The Commission represented government, employers, trade unions and other interests, including education. In 1983 it had still not fallen foul of the new conviction politics, and its proposal for a YTS had the support of all sides of industry and all the UK's main political parties (Manpower Services Commission 1981a, 1981b). This scheme was not a product of 'New Right' ideology.

The problem that the YTS was intended to solve once and for all was that Britain's education and training systems were not equally useful for all young people. Education was seen as serving the needs of young people with academic aptitude. They could succeed in the main examinations for 16-year-olds (GCE O-levels at the time), proceed to A-levels and then to degrees. With their talent certified, they stood excellent chances of finding employers who would offer them jobs with status, training, above-average pay and career prospects. Other young people were being turned into early failures. By the age of 16 there was nowhere further for them to go within mainstream education, and this remained the case despite the replacement of grammar schools and secondary moderns by comprehensives in most parts of the country.

One response to this problem would have been to dilute the academic bias in school curricula; another would have been to create alternative technical or vocational tracks. The latter was in fact the intention when technical and modern secondary schools began to open between the World Wars and when, after 1944, they became part of a national system of tripartite secondary education. Since 1986 there have been renewed efforts to create vocational tracks geared to National Vocational Qualifications (NVQs) and, in particular, General National Vocational Qualifications (GNVQs). However, up to now all such efforts have been balked by a determination in some quarters, inside and outside education, to defend traditional academic standards and, related to this, the low status that has blighted vocational courses and qualifications. In 1983 the view that prevailed was that education was so much part of the problem that it could not be central in its solution.

Some young people who left school at 16 fared reasonably well. They obtained jobs with training – sometimes with day release, which allowed them to continue their education – and could expect to progress to skilled status and perhaps beyond. In some of these jobs training was organised within formal apprenticeship schemes. 'The problem' was said to be that around a third of all young people left school at 16 without any useful qualifications, then entered jobs (if they obtained any) which offered no systematic training or opportunities for continuing education, and time was not eroding the size of this group. Some industries that had offered substantial numbers of apprenticeships were in long-term decline in terms of the size of their work-force, if not of output. Engineering was the leading example. And in the early 1980s around a fifth of all manufacturing jobs were being lost in the deepest recession since the Second World War. Moreover, the structural changes in the UK economy and labour markets since the early 1970s had created a mass youth unemployment problem. The answer, it was believed, was a national training scheme which would offer all 16- and 17-year-old school-leavers the opportunity to acquire vocational skills and worthwhile qualifications. This was seen as necessary not just for the young people's good, but also for the economy. The proportion of low-level jobs was known to be in long-term decline, while the proportion of high-level jobs was increasing. A new technological revolution was in progress, the micro-electronic information-processing and communications revolution, and there were fears of Britain failing to produce the kind of skilled work-force that would be needed.

It would have been possible to call the intended solution a national apprenticeship scheme. However, at the time (the early 1980s) those responsible wanted to avoid some features of traditional apprenticeships – especially the practice of treating as skilled all individuals who simply 'served their time', irrespective of their actual competence – and also to avoid the manner in which apprentice training separated skilled from unskilled labour. The YTS was intended to provide all young people with opportunities to become skilled, albeit to different levels.

The German apprenticeship system was the model. In Germany virtually all young people were, and still are, either trained as skilled workers within the dual system (on-the-job training combined with continuing education) or achieve the academic qualifications needed to enter higher education. Its skilled work-force has been widely seen as a major asset to the German economy and a reason for its outstanding post-war growth record. Asserting that nearly all young people in Germany become skilled invites questions about who does the unskilled jobs. The answer is that skilled German workers do not necessarily obtain commensurate employment. Females, in particular, have tended to be tracked towards low-status and low-paid occupations. Also, since the Second World War Germany has hosted pools of unskilled migrant labour. Even so, the German system has given virtually all young people the feeling of accomplishing something worthwhile, and employers have rarely complained of skill shortages. Britain's YTS was intended to replicate these achievements.

It may be worth stressing that the problem that the YTS was designed to address was not a general lack of opportunities for young people from working-class backgrounds, nor a general low rate of upward mobility into higher-level occupations. Most people in Britain's managerial and professional jobs are recruited from beneath. The typical working-class family with two children can expect at least one to experience upward mobility (see Goldthorpe *et al.* 1987). Modern Britain has never been marked by especially strong or impenetrable class divisions. The 'problem' that YTS addressed involved those school-leavers who were not being offered opportunities to acquire further recognised skills and qualifications.

THE SOLUTION

During the five years up to 1983 the MSC had operated a Youth Opportunities Programme (YOP). This had been hastily designed and introduced in 1978 to address an unpredicted and unwelcome problem of mass youth unemployment. Following the oil price spirals of the early and mid-1970s unemployment had soared, especially among school-leavers. Many were stranded in a situation where they were unable to gain even work experience because they could not obtain employment, and their lack of experience made them unattractive to employers. YOP was designed to break this cycle by, in most cases, giving otherwise unemployed young people up to six months' work experience either with an employer or on a community or workshop-based project. YOP was designed to deal with a temporary problem, and the legislation allowed the programme to operate for only five years. By then, so it was believed in 1978, the economy would have strengthened, unemployment would be disappearing, and the demographic tide (the rising numbers in successive school-leaving cohorts during the 1970s) would have turned (Manpower Services Commission 1977). In the event, unemployment was even higher by 1983, more young people than in 1978 needed to be accommodated on YOP, and when they left the programme the majority were becoming unemployed.

In 1983 the MSC stressed that the YTS would be an entirely different kind of measure. It was not meant to be just another temporary 'band aid' but was intended to be permanent. It was introduced as just the initial step in a 'New Training Initiative'. The MSC insisted that the measure was not primarily a response to unemployment but was a training scheme first and foremost. YTS was made available for all young people, employed and unemployed, and employers were invited to register their young employees as well as taking on additional trainees. Unlike YOP, YTS was to offer quality training on and off the job, initially lasting at least one year, leading to worthwhile qualifications. All 16- and 17-year-olds who were otherwise unemployed were to be guaranteed places, and this guarantee was generally met throughout the scheme's lifetime. But YTS was not targeted at just the tail end: the intention was that all young people recruited by employers at the age of 16 or 17 would become involved. The aim was to make the entire work-force trained and skilled, like Germany's. In most cases the extra training was to be provided by employers (Mode A), but other provisions (Mode B) were possible where there was a shortfall in employer-based provision, and for young people whose special needs required training that employers could not offer. YTS was not designed mainly for the exceptionally disadvantaged, though it was believed that such young people – those who previously were the least likely to be trained, who included girls and ethnic-minority youth – would derive the greatest benefit. Equal opportunities, meaning access to all provisions irrespective of race and sex, were enshrined in the scheme's regulations. All training providers were required to operate equal opportunities.

EARLY SUCCESS

Throughout the 1980s government statements consistently hailed YTS as a huge success. The launch was certainly successful. The new scheme had to be sold to young people and to employers. Firms had to be persuaded to create places which school-leavers had to be persuaded to accept. Up to 1988 young people had the options of staying in full-time education, finding proper jobs if they could, or registering as unemployed and claiming benefit. The MSC was remarkably successful with both groups. Most large companies and thousands of smaller firms became involved. Thus it was possible from 1983 onwards for YTS to be the most common next step for 16-year-old school-leavers. The initial appeal of the new measure among young people was indicated by an immediate drop in the stay-on rate in full-time education from 45 per cent to 42 per cent. This in fact became a point of criticism: YTS was encouraging young people to quit full-time education prematurely. Educators sometimes complained that otherwise unemployed young people who entered YTS received allowances, and even those who remained unemployed received social security, whereas full-time students were paid nothing (though their parents were eligible for Child Benefit).

In the early years of YTS it was possible to draw favourable comparisons with young people's experiences on YOP. On YTS more were receiving 'real training' and obtaining qualifications. Needless to say, it was always recognised that it would be impossible to turn out fully skilled workers in just one year. However, the one-year scheme that was launched in 1983 was just the first stage. This led to the second stage in 1986, when the normal length of YTS was extended to two years. Once again, everyone realised that training for many occupations required more than two years. The hope, when YTS was introduced, was that after their year (subsequently two years) within the scheme young people would progress into employment in which their training would continue.

One reason why employer recruitment was successful when YTS was launched was the fairly generous funding that was then available (see Raggatt 1988). Trainees' allowances were fully covered, plus most of the additional costs that trainers had to incur. However, it was no-one's intention that, in the longer term, the state should fund all training in industry. From 1986 onwards financial support for trainers became less generous, especially in year two. The MSC wanted to double the normal length of training without doubling its own costs. Employers were expected to contribute to the costs of training; after all, they would benefit from the supply of skilled labour. The generous funding early on was meant to kick-start the initiative. Employers were expected, in time, to accept greater responsibility for the costs of initial and, to an even greater extent, their employees' continuing training.

During the 1980s this appeared to happen. Firms created training departments, managers and budgets, and the proportion of employees receiving training increased (this is monitored regularly in the quarterly *Labour Force Survey*). Training gained a stronger profile. Firms began to sign up for Department of Employment recognition as 'Investors in People'. Health and safety legislation, and a broader enthusiasm for 'total quality management', also boosted spending on, and the profile of, formal training. YTS itself was promoted strenuously through newspaper and television advertising which featured blue chip companies such as Wimpey, and even Bobby Robson, the England soccer manager.

WHAT WENT WRONG?

Hindsight is always invaluable, and there is no implication in what follows that the problems that beset the YTS should have been foreseen in 1983. It is important to analyse what went wrong, not so as to apportion blame but so as to learn lessons and avoid further policy failures.

The context of unemployment

Whatever the MSC said about YTS being a training scheme first and foremost, the plain fact was that the scheme was launched amidst the highest unemployment ever recorded in Britain. It was probably inevitable that many members of the public, including young people, would see the scheme first and foremost as an alternative to joblessness. However often the MSC stressed that YTS was fundamentally different, it did take over from YOP, which had been designed to tackle youth unemployment, and attitudes towards the earlier measure were always likely to be transferred onto its successor scheme (see Raffe 1987).

It is equally pertinent that YTS never eliminated straightforward youth employment. This was never made illegal. In fact, between 1982 and 1988 the government had other measures – the Young Workers Scheme, and then the New Workers Scheme – which subsidised firms that recruited unemployed young people irrespective of whether they received any training, provided their pay was beneath a ceiling. There were several reasons why many firms preferred to employ young people even though they could have obtained them free on YTS, and the subsidies available on the parallel schemes were not the most important. First, employers knew that by offering proper jobs they could take their pick of school-leavers. Second, some did not want the inconvenience and form-filling, or to have to tailor their training to YTS regulations. They regarded the subsidies that were available as trivial in relation to their total labour costs. Third, in some industries the trade unions had objections to trainees on allowances replacing employees on negotiated rates of pay. The outcome was that, throughout the 1980s, it remained possible for school-leavers to look for jobs, and in the parts of Britain where unemployment was relatively low there were always more jobs than YTS places (see Banks *et al.* 1992). School-leavers would first look for jobs, and would consider schemes only if their job-searching proved unsuccessful. Jobs were seen as preferable in every respect. The pay was better, there were usually better prospects of long-term positions, and the training could be just as thorough and useful. Just as young people regarded YTS as second best to employment, it was probably inevitable that employers would regard youth trainees as individuals who had been unable to find real jobs. The glossy brochures and television adverts never spoke for most of the scheme's users.

Types of schemes

The MSC distinguished only between employer-led and other schemes, but young people soon realised that there were other differences. They distinguished between good and bad schemes. Researchers who tracked young people's experiences were able to construct typologies that distinguished various types and degrees of goodness and badness (see Lee *et al.* 1989; Raffe 1987; Roberts and Parsell 1992).

First, there were schemes which employers used as the initial stage in longer training programmes. When recruiting to these YTS places, the employers often restricted their intakes to the numbers that they intended to retain for the full programmes and then absorb into their work-forces. David Raffe (1987) described such schemes as a 'sponsorship' sector of YTS. The employers usually restricted recruitment to the numbers they hoped to employ partly because their firms would often spend in excess of the MSC contribution on such schemes, and partly because they wanted the recruits to feel part of the businesses from the outset. Young people on such schemes were sometimes granted employee status, and paid in excess of the basic allowance, from day one.

Second, there were 'youth try-out schemes', described as a 'contest' sector by David Raffe. On such schemes the employers would use the training period to assess potential recruits. At the end of the training, if not before, the employers would pick the best and discard the rest.

Third, there were cases where employers used the YTS to create 'low-paid youth jobs' – office junior and shop assistant's assistant for example. It was on such schemes that young people were most likely to complain of being treated as 'slave labour'. Some found that their training involved doing much the same work as employees but for considerably less pay. Such trainees could be retained as employees if vacancies arose at the right time, or if they had demonstrated such proficiency as to be considered indispensable. However, it was also possible for employers to use YTS as a never-ending source of incredibly cheap temporary labour.

Fourth, there were some schemes where young people stood little chance of being retained but which equipped them with skills, qualifications or experience which stood them in good stead on returning to external labour markets. David Raffe (1987) described such schemes as a 'credentialling' sector. There were some clear examples – schemes that offered training in office and computer skills were the best – but such schemes were a tiny proportion of all YTS places. However, if young people derived long-term benefits from their training this was usually as a result of being kept-on. Those who returned to external labour markets generally found that the experience, skills and qualifications acquired during their training carried little weight when approaching employers (Roberts and Parsell 1992); they had the countervailing handicap of having been trained and then discarded.

Fifth, some schemes seemed to confer no benefits except by 'warehousing' young people, temporarily keeping them off the streets and unemployment registers. Many Mode B schemes appeared to fall into this category. By 1986 the MSC had realised that Mode B seemed to be officially designating these schemes as second-class. Subsequently this terminology was dropped – official statements referred to employer-led and other training, or basic and premium places – but across the country this did not prevent young people and their families continuing to talk of 'rubbish schemes'.

With hindsight it is easy to recognise the inevitability of YTS operating in different ways in different places. A strength of the scheme was that in most cases young people were trained by, and on the premises of, employers. The YTS was not a network of dedicated training centres. Given that thousands of separate employers were, in a sense, 'franchised' to run the scheme, how the YTS worked in practice was bound to vary according to what each firm was able and willing to offer (see Chandler and Wallace 1990). The national adverts referred to *the* YTS, whereas young people spoke of doing *a* YTS. The popular schemes, generally the sponsorship variety, were able to be selective about who was recruited; reasonable school-leaving qualifications were usually required. At the bottom of the league there were 'sink schemes', generally in the 'warehousing sector', that took otherwise unwanted young people, most of whom faced subsequent unemployment.

These differences between schemes became wider as local reputations were established, and especially in the late-1980s, when trainers were required to part-fund the schemes. Employers who themselves stood much of the cost became increasingly careful to train only young people who were likely to prove worthwhile investments (Lee *et al.* 1989). Other schemes cut back to basics, and frills, such as adventure courses, were axed. Off-the-job training was brought in-house, rather than purchased from further education colleges. Community projects were expected to place trainees with firms for part of the programmes and to raise employer contributions to the costs of training. This led to the 'rent-a-trainee' regime. The least advantaged young people, who were supposed to derive the greatest benefit, became the least likely to profit from the YTS.

Everyone griped about money. Throughout the lifetime of YTS trainees complained about their 'derisory' allowances. Many trainers complained that the scheme was under-funded. However, the young people felt badly rewarded only when they took young workers, rather than full-time students, as their reference group, and – as explained earlier – it had never been the intention, nor were there any demands from business, for the state to accept financial responsibility for all industry-based training. The government funding was always sufficient to maintain places for all eligible young people. And unemployment was so detested that most young people were willing to enter programmes that offered literally 'anything better than the dole'. It was not state under-funding that undermined the YTS.

The academic yardstick

Overarching everything, YTS had the problem that the experience, skills and qualifications that it offered could not match the appeal of academic credentials. It was known that the best-qualified 16-year-olds tended to remain in full-time education, and that those entering the YTS were generally less able academically. The qualifications gained by young people who stayed on the academic route – A-levels, then degrees – were long-established, well-known and highly regarded by employers. YTS was no match.

It has proved difficult to establish exactly what employers want of young people. If given the opportunity, some will complain about virtually everything – their appearance, attitudes, standards of reading, writing and arithmetic, and, of course, their vocational inexperience (see Dench 1993; Hunt and Small 1981). The knee-jerk reaction of many employers has been to express approval of any course with technical or vocational in the title. However, the Queen's English Society has been able to produce survey evidence showing that what employers really want is better communication skills (Lamb 1994). Predictably, a survey commissioned by the Business and Technology Education Council found that employers were particularly keen for recruits to have more vocational skills (Quentin Bell Organisation 1995). However, as far as career opportunities are concerned, what employers say is less important than what they actually do, and in hiring situations it is academic qualifications that have always carried the greatest weight. Throughout the 1980s academic attainments remained far and away the best predictors of how young people's careers would develop. All other credentials were devalued in comparison (see Banks *et al.* 1992; Bennett *et al.* 1992).

Employers are more likely to be impressed when vocational qualifications are offered as well as, rather than in lieu of, academic attainments. Once individuals are in employment, vocational qualifications can help them to get ahead, but in getting started it is academic qualifications that continue to count most. YTS became the base of an alternative route towards qualifications and employment but one which never earned even near equal status to the academic track. One suspects that this was always anticipated by those who designed YTS. It bore many of the hallmarks of being intended for other people's children.

FRAYING EDGES

The high tide of YTS, certainly in terms of numbers, was reached soon after it became a two year scheme in 1986. Shortly after then the scheme began to fray on several edges.

Education preferred

From the mid-1980s the educational stay-on rate of 16-year-olds resumed its pre-1983 climb. During the early 1990s it reached 70 per cent. By then, a quarter of the age group had shifted into full-time education since 1983, and YTS was the main loser. This was the principal reason, exacerbated by the declining size of 16-year-old cohorts, for the fall in the numbers entering YTS. This enabled the MSC to cull the weakest, least popular and (conveniently) also the most expensive schemes: training which was not employer-based was not viable without premium funding. If all other things had remained equal the cull might have strengthened the YTS overall, but the trend towards young people remaining in education made this impossible. Young people were giving YTS the thumbs down. They seemed to have got the message that academic courses and qualifications gave the best vocational returns, and they were willing to sacrifice the training allowance available on YTS. In many cases this was no hardship. Many students earned more in evening and weekend jobs (see Hutson and Cheung 1991), and the lifestyle and status of the student were more appealing than becoming a trainee. YTS was unable to compete. The haemorrhage out of YTS was mainly by the 16-year-olds who had previously made up the better-qualified entrants. By the end of the 1980s YTS was looking distinctly residual. Around two-thirds of 16-year-olds were continuing in full-time education; some of the remainder obtained proper jobs; YTS took most of the rest.

As its intake declined in size and academic quality the proportions of youth trainees gaining qualifications on the scheme, and progressing directly into employment, began to decline (*Labour Market Quarterly Report* August 1993). It was difficult to disentangle the contribution of the rising level of general unemployment across the country from 1990 onwards from that of the declining quality of trainees, but there was a further tarnishing of YT's public image. By the early 1990s YT (as it then was) appeared to be in an irreversible cycle of decline.

Status zero

It was never possible to establish whether there was a post-1983 rise in the number of 'refuseniks' opting for unemployment and declining to enter YTS, but their existence gained a higher profile. They were always a small minority, well below 10 per cent of the age group, but their behaviour provoked outrage from Government ministers and the popular press. They were the principal reason given for withdrawing most unemployed 16- and 17-year-olds' entitlement to social security benefits in 1988 – since when youth unemployment has officially ceased to exist. However, there have continued to be 'status zero' young people: those not in education, training or employment. A 1990s study in South Glamorgan (Istance *et al.* 1994) found that at any time around 17 per cent of 16- and 17-year-olds were status zero. Most occupied this status only for brief periods, but around 7 per cent of the age group appeared permanently lost. Some of these were effectively becoming status zero before being eligible to leave full-time education – they were irregular attenders during their final years of compulsory schooling.

Researchers who have questioned young people who appear to prefer unemployment to education or training have found that very few have any principled objections to becoming more highly trained or educated. The majority have been disillusioned by their prior experiences of training, and education also in many cases (see Aspire Consultants 1996; Wilkinson 1995). They see no point in rejoining the 'black magic roundabout' of schemes which lead only to 'rubbish jobs' or back to unemployment. Maybe it was not the cause, but YTS was vulnerable to criticism for failing to prevent the development of a youth underclass or, to use European Union terminology, excluded groups.

The end of consensus

The withdrawal of unemployed 16- and 17-year-olds' benefit entitlement in 1988 was one of the straws that broke the trade union movement's willingness to endorse government programmes for the unemployed. A wide body of trade union opinion had always been concerned that trainees might be substituted for, or would undercut and undermine the pay of, employees. The TUC had always insisted that participation in government programmes should be voluntary. In 1988 the trade union representatives withdrew from the MSC, which proved a death sentence for that body. Maybe the government welcomed the opportunity to cull the MSC. Government thinking had drifted well away from the MSC's corporatist, consensual style.

As an interim measure the MSC was replaced by a Training Commission – composed of representatives of all the old interest groups, minus the trade unions – which assumed responsibility for the former MSC's training programmes. Before long this Commission had been replaced by a Training Agency taking instructions directly from the Department of Employment. In 1990 this Agency was re-absorbed as a division within the Employment

Department. These administrative changes were partly the cause and partly the symptoms of declining public confidence in YTS and other government programmes.

Consolidating low standards

YTS always had critics who accused the scheme of concealing unemployment (depressing the figures), offering just a temporary palliative for joblessness, and depressing wage levels and expectations (see Finn 1987; Rees and Atkinson 1982). By the end of the 1980s the grounds for criticism had widened. A particularly wounding accusation was that the scheme was not tackling the poorly trained and qualified condition of Britain's work-force but consolidating it. In the early years it had been credible to envisage YTS gradually upgrading Britain's workers, but by the end of the 1980s standards on the scheme were clearly stagnating or even declining. Most young people who passed through the scheme left with low-level skills which equipped them for semi-skilled jobs at best, and most of the qualifications earned by trainees were low-level ones. The scheme was vulnerable to accusations of equipping twenty-first-century Britain with a low-grade work-force (see Ashton et al. 1989).

Attention was drawn to the fact that the proportion of young people achieving no qualifications whatsoever, and admitting difficulties with such basic skills as reading, writing and arithmetic, was not declining but remained at roughly the same level as in the 1970s: around one in ten. There had been an overall rise in levels of educational attainment, but the very weakest young people had not been part of this trend (see Ekinsmyth and Bynner 1994). Rather than catching up, the least advantaged young people had been dropping further behind.

Maybe it was only to be expected that, by the end of the 1980s, most scheme managers would be anything but keen to recruit less able young people, or those who were reluctant to accept places. By then many of the original schemes with social objectives, and predictably low success rates, had been axed. Moreover, Government funding had become dependent on filled places, which meant that, in order to maximise their incomes, scheme organisers needed to recruit young people who would 'stay the course'. When, in the 1990s, funding began to be geared to outcomes expressed in terms of the numbers gaining qualifications at stipulated levels, scheme managers' preference for at least reasonably able and motivated recruits would have strengthened (comparable pressures are believed to have led to the rise in the numbers of pupils excluded from LEA schools). There was an irony in pressures to raise or maintain standards on YTS increasing the vulnerability of the highly disadvantaged groups of young people for whom special measures – the antecedents of YTS in the 1970s – had originally been designed.

Unequal opportunities

A further set of criticisms was that YTS was failing to deliver equal opportunities. Ethnic-minority youth tended to be clustered on the schemes with the poorest employment prospects (Connolly *et al.* 1991; Cross and Smith 1987). Most boys and girls were trained in traditionally masculine and feminine occupations (Cockburn 1987).

YTS managers could claim, with some justification, that these criticisms were unfair. The YTS could hardly hope to override all the historical and socio-economic processes responsible for the inequalities between Britain's ethnic groups. And young people entered the scheme with career aspirations that were already gendered. Trainers knew that girls were most likely to obtain employment in which they would settle if they were equipped to compete for women's jobs, and similarly with boys. It would have been equally reasonable to point out that no country's education and training has managed to avoid a minority, usually between 10 and 20 per cent of the age group, failing to reach its basic grade; this applies even in Germany. However, the reasonableness of such disclaimers did not prevent the criticisms contributing to weakening the YTS.

YOUTH TRAINING IN THE 1990s

During the 1990s there were two attempts to relaunch and revive the YTS. Neither worked, but both reduced the scheme's visibility and central government's responsibility for its implementation.

Training and Enterprise Councils (TECs)

In 1990 responsibility for the implementation of Youth Training (as the measure was retitled) was transferred to local TECs in England

and Wales, and to LECs (Local Enterprise Companies) in Scotland. TECs and LECs are organised like private companies, with boards of directors, mostly local employers. They have contracts with central government to implement a range of employment and training programmes in their areas. The TECs and LECs then sub-contract most of this work to local training providers. The aim of this devolution has been to make the relevant policies and programmes more responsive to local conditions, especially the needs of local employers (see Coffield 1992). An inevitable corollary has been that how national programmes actually operate has become more varied than ever. As regards YT, the basic allowances for trainees remained the same throughout the country, but the enti-tlements of training providers and the requirements placed upon them became more diverse. Matters depended on how a local TEC decided to spend its income so as to meet its own contractual obli-gations. After 1990, if any business or individual felt aggrieved at how YT was being run, there was no point in complaining to a Government minister; the correspondence would be directed to the TEC. Public awareness of the TECs and their programmes has never matched the profile achieved by the MSC and its measures in the 1980s. Since then school education has been a more prominent national issue, due largely to the 'nationalisation' of the curriculum and testing.

Youth Credits

In 1991 the Employment Department began to pilot Youth Credits and then spread them gradually throughout the country. As Youth Credits became available, the title Youth Training was allowed to lapse. The credit system gives the 'purchaser', the young person, a voucher with a money value (usually around £1,000) which can be used to buy approved training, and training providers are expected to compete to attract customers. The aim is to increase the purchaser's sense of responsibility for his or her own career devel-opment and to individualise responsibility for failure to obtain useful training. However, a major problem facing would-be purchasers of Youth Training in the early 1990s was that the credit system could not, of itself, widen the choice that was on offer (see Felstead 1993; MacDonald and Coffield 1993). It was the same problem as that involved in extending parents' choice of schools: not everyone can be admitted to the most popular establishments.

By 1995 Youth Credits had spread nation-wide but with little public debate. This was partly because of their gradual introduction, and partly because their distribution and administration was (and still is) handled by the TECs, which are allowed to attach their own brand names to the vouchers. A 'big bang' will occur if and when young people are empowered to use their credits to purchase either education in schools or colleges or training with employers or other training providers – or if and when the most popular establishments are allowed to charge top-up fees. In the early 1990s the behaviour of young people did not change when Youth Credits were introduced in their areas (Croxford *et al.* 1996; Employment Department 1992). Most young people and employers expressed general approval but the appeal of the credits did not attract young people out of full-time education and into training. However, slightly more training was drawn into the Government scheme. It appeared that when young people holding vouchers with a money value began applying to employers, businesses that were able to qualify took the necessary steps to obtain reimbursement from their TECs.

ALTERNATIVE MEASURES

Vocational qualifications

By the mid-1990s the remnants of YTS had become a backwater. Government efforts to improve young people's opportunities and to raise the skills of Britain's work-force were being channelled into education.

In 1986 the Department of Employment had created a National Council of Vocational Qualifications. Its brief was to impose order on the 'jungle' of vocational credentials, thereby increasing their value to employers and employees, raising their status and broadening their appeal. The Council set about this task by creating a framework of five levels within which existing and new qualifications could be located. Simultaneously 'lead bodies' representing different industries were established to specify the competencies required at each level. The idea was that NVQs would differ from previous qualifications in certifying what individuals could actually do, rather than merely what they knew. Putting employers in charge (they dominated all the lead bodies) was intended to guarantee that the qualifications would certify useful skills, which would therefore be recognised and used by employers and would therefore appeal to trainees. NVQs are designed primarily for people in jobs or employer-based training. Most of the instruction and testing can be in work situations. An initial idea was that youth (and adult) trainees would be able to work towards NVQs, which, it was hoped, would strengthen the appeal of the training. In the event the advent of NVQs did not reverse the decline of the YTS.

During the 1990s a parallel set of general vocational qualifications (GNVQs) was introduced. These are meant to be relevant in broad fields of employment, rather than specific industries and occupations, and are normally gained through college-based study. These qualifications proved an immediate hit. There was a rapid take-up in further education colleges and many schools, and massive enrolments by 16- and 17-year-olds, especially the attainment bands for whom three A-levels were considered inappropriate. However, the government wanted to avoid these new qualifications being regarded as inferior to academic credentials and declared that a Level 3 GNVQ was the equivalent of 2 A-levels.

By the early 1990s the Employment Department was setting targets for improving the quality of Britain's supply of labour in terms of the numbers to achieve qualifications at different levels. Within a few years some of the targets were being met, or even exceeded, as a result of the rising enrolments by young people in full-time education, and of the rising numbers who were achieving qualifications – mainly A-levels and GNVQs (Department for Education and Employment 1996). Contrary to the intention in 1983, the targets were being met not through the strengthening and enlargement of employer-based routes but through full-time study in schools and colleges. This was part of the case for the merger of the Employment Department and the Department for Education which happened in 1995.

Modern Apprenticeships

In 1995 Modern Apprenticeships were introduced to operate alongside Youth Training/Credits. This new initiative was an attempt to revive the flagging workplace route to skills, qualifications and career opportunities. For these purposes the term 'apprenticeship' was officially rehabilitated; it had never lost its appeal in industry or among school-leavers.

Modern Apprenticeships are aimed at young people who have

achieved, or are judged capable of achieving, A-levels or their vocational equivalent. All the apprentices are expected to reach this level. Sixteen- and seventeen-year-old Modern Apprentices purchase their training with Youth Credits, and may receive just the mandatory training allowance, though in practice the majority are given employee status and paid wages, just like traditional apprentices. Older school and college leavers can also start Modern Apprenticeships, funded from the TECs' Youth Credit budgets. A benefit for employers whose training receives Modern Apprenticeship accreditation, apart from the cash value of the Youth Credit, is to make the positions easily understood and attractive to applicants. Sixteen- and seventeen-year-old school-leavers who do not seek or obtain Modern Apprenticeships (or employment) have continued to be able to use their Youth Credits to 'purchase' more conventional forms of Youth Training.

By the time that Modern Apprenticeships were up and running there had been an almost total reversal of the 1983 priorities. The main growth area in the vocational preparation of 16–18-year-olds had not been employer-based but school- and college-based. The beneficiaries of increased government spending in the age group had not been those who were least advantaged but the high- and middle-ranking academic achievers who were remaining in full-time education until 18 to take A-levels or GNVQs, and who, in the 1990s, were progressing into Modern Apprenticeships or an enlarged university system in unprecedented numbers.

THE FUTURE

The Dearing Report (Dearing 1996) has taken much of the normal hazard out of forecasting. During the 1990s Sir Ron Dearing became the Department for Education's most reliable trouble-shooter, able to achieve consensus on formerly controversial topics such as the National Curriculum and educational testing. In 1996 he did it again with a report on qualifications for 16–19-year-olds which was greeted with bipartisan enthusiasm. His recommendations included, first, a common framework for all qualifications (with four levels, from entry to advanced) which would certify the equivalence of academic and vocational courses, and, second, the replacement of Youth Training by National Traineeships which could lead into Modern Apprenticeships. If such proposals are to be implemented there are several lessons from YTS that can usefully be borne in mind.

First, a common framework which decrees the equivalence of academic and vocational courses will not guarantee their treatment in this way in the wider society. Although it was all Youth Training, young people distinguished the good schemes from the bad. The leaving certificates that all trainees were awarded were never as important as the other qualifications (if any) that were listed on them. The same may happen to a future National Diploma; those listing A-levels may be regarded as better than those listing NVQs or GNVQs. Governments do not have the final say in these matters. This rests with the admissions policies of educational institutions, employers' recruitment and promotion practices, and the views of young people and their parents.

Second, policies and provisions for the 16–19 age group create hostages to fortune if they pledge themselves to 'tougher' versions of equal opportunities. Given all that has already happened to children in their homes and schools, it is highly improbable the benefits of 16–19 provisions will be distributed regardless of gender, ethnic and social class backgrounds.

Third, any drive to raise standards risks sacrificing the weakest. This happened with YT, when trainers were given a financial interest in dealing with young people who they knew could be made employer-ready and who could be relied on to achieve qualifications. There will be the same risks in making A-levels or Level 3 GNVQs or NVQs the targets for all provisions.

Fourth, despite all the talk of the economy needing a more highly qualified and skilled work-force, roughly a quarter of all jobs are still non-skilled manual. Education and training which leads into such jobs will never be upgraded in anyone's eyes without upgrading the occupations themselves, and the actual trend since the 1970s has been in the opposite direction.

Fifth, unemployment cannot be ignored. If substantial numbers of students or trainees exit into unemployment, the reputations of their schemes and courses will always be blighted. The status of any programme depends less on what happens during it than on what happens on exit and on the recruits it attracts. We now know from experience in the 1980s that making young people better qualified is insufficient to generate a demand for their labour. Most measures work best (for workers at any rate) in conditions of full employment. Most types of education and training satisfy virtually everyone who is able to progress into commensurate occupations. Full employment is certainly the best-known way of improving the life chances of the least advantaged young people. They have the option of being able to move rapidly to adult earnings without artificial delays. Their terms and conditions of employment strengthen when labour demand is strong, closing the gap with the more highly skilled. Training and education are unlikely to be as effective, and are always likely to be regarded as poor substitutes for proper jobs unless operating alongside full employment policies.

REFERENCES

Ashton, D.N., Maguire, M.J., and Spilsbury, M. (1989) *Restructuring the Labour Market: The Implications for Youth*, London: Macmillan.

Aspire Consultants (1996) *Disaffection and Non-Participation in Education, Training and Employment by Individuals Aged 18–20*, London: Department for Education and Employment.

Banks, M., Bates, I., Breakwell, G., Bynner, J., Emler, N., Jamieson, L. and Roberts, K. (1992) *Careers and Identities*, Milton Keynes: Open University Press.

Bennett, R., Glennerster, H. and Nevison, D. (1992) *Investing in Skill: Expected Returns to Vocational Studies*, Discussion Paper WSP/83, London: London School of Economics.

Chandler, J. and Wallace, C. (1990) 'Some alternatives in youth training: Franchise and corporatist models', in D. Gleeson (ed.) *Training and its Alternatives*, Milton Keynes: Open University Press.

Cockburn, C. (1987) *Two Track Training*, London: Macmillan.

Coffield, F. (1992) 'Training and Enterprise Councils: The last throw of voluntarism?' *Policy Studies*, 13(4): 11–32.

Connolly, M., Roberts, K., Ben-Tovim, G. and Torkington, P. (1991) *Black Youth in Liverpool*, Culemborg: Giordano Bruno.

Cross, M., and Smith, D.I. (eds) (1987) *Black Youth Futures*, Leicester: National Youth Bureau.

Croxford, L., Raffe, D. and Surridge, P. (1996) *The Impact of Youth Credits*, University of Edinburgh: Centre for Educational Sociology.

Dearing, R. (1996) *Review of Qualifications for 16–19 Year Olds*, Sheffield: Department for Education and Employment.

Dench, S. (1993) 'What types of people are employers seeking to employ?', paper presented to Employment Department/Policy Studies Institute conference on *Unemployment in Focus*, Rotherham.

Department for Education and Employment (1996) *Labour Market and Skill Trends 1996/1997*, Sheffield.

Ekinsmyth, C. and Bynner, J. (1994) *The Basic Skills of Young Adults*, London: Adult Literacy and Basic Skills Unit.

Employment Department (1992) *Training Credits: A Report on the First 12 Months*, London.

Felstead, A. (1993) *Putting Individuals in Charge: Leaving Skills Behind?* University of Leicester: Department of Sociology, Discussion Paper S93/9.

Finn, D. (1987) *Training Without Jobs*, London: Macmillan.

Goldthorpe, J.H., Llewellyn, C. and Payne, C. (1987) *Social Mobility and Class Structure in Modern Britain*, Oxford: Clarendon Press.

Hunt, J. and Small, P. (1981) *Employing Young People*, Edinburgh: Scottish Council for Research in Education.

Hutson, S. and Cheung, W. (1991), 'Saturday jobs: Sixth formers in the labour market and the family', in C. Marsh and S. Arber (eds) *Family and Household: Division and Change*, London: Macmillan.

Istance, D., Rees, G. and Williamson, H. (1994) *Young People not in Education, Training or Employment*, Cardiff: South Glamorgan Training and Enterprise Council.

Lamb, B.C. (1994) *A National Survey of Communication Skills of Young Entrants to Industry and Commerce*, London: Queen's English Society.

Lee, D.J., Marsden, D., Rickman, P. and Duncombe, J. (1989) *Scheming for Youth: A Study of YTS in the Enterprise Culture*, Milton Keynes: Open University Press.

MacDonald, R. and Coffield, F. (1993) 'Young people and training credits: An early exploration', *British Journal of Education and Work* 6: 5–21.

Manpower Services Commission (1977) *Young People and Work*, London.

—— (1981a) *A New Training Initiative: a Consultative Document*, London.

—— (1981b) *A New Training Initiative: An Agenda for Action*, London.

Quentin Bell Organisation (1995) *Skilless Youth Costs Britain Millions*, London: press release.

Raffe, D. (1987) 'The context of the Youth Training Scheme: An analysis of its strategy and development', *British Journal of Education and Work* 1: 1–33.

Raggatt, P. (1988) 'Quality control in the dual system of West Germany', *Oxford Review of Education* 14: 163–86.

Rees, T.L. and Atkinson, P. (eds) (1982) *Youth Unemployment and State Intervention*, London: Routledge.

Roberts, K. and Parsell, G. (1992) 'The stratification of Youth Training', *British Journal of Education and Work* 5: 65–83.

Wilkinson, C. (1995) *The Dropout Society*, Leicester: Youth Work Press.

Chapter 6

Youth homelessness
Marginalising the marginalised?

Susan Hutson and Mark Liddiard

INTRODUCTION

Young homeless people are perhaps the most explicit and distasteful indictment of growing inequalities in the UK. Young people living and sleeping on the streets and in insecure accommodation are hardly congruent with the notion of a 'classless society'. In this chapter, we examine youth homelessness to illustrate the quite spurious nature of claims that the UK is moving towards a 'classless society'. In particular, we highlight the general discrimination against youth by society and social policy and the more specific discrimination against poorer and more disadvantaged young people, such as those who are unemployed and homeless.

The chapter falls into two parts. In the first part, specific policies are set against general trends. The increase in youth homelessness since the early 1980s is often blamed on a number of Conservative policies such as the restructuring of welfare benefits in 1988 and the run-down of council housing. In this chapter, these are placed in the broader context of trends in the labour and housing markets which have seen young people become increasingly marginalised, a process which has been compounded by the Government's restructuring of welfare benefits for unemployed young people, which has significantly contributed to the rise in youth homelessness in the UK. However, broad trends in the labour market can reflect more than national economic policies, and may ultimately be subservient to international and even global economic developments. In this sense, one could argue that a General Election and a change of government may bring little change to the plight of the homeless in the UK.

The second part of the chapter looks in more detail at the manner in which young homeless people have been increasingly marginalised – not simply by legislation, but also in terms of policy responses, research and even the media. For example, the response to youth homelessness is in terms of special projects rather than youth policies. The 1989 Children Act delivers services only to care-leavers, rather than to young people more broadly disadvantaged. Current research on youth homelessness stresses the importance of dysfunctional families, while the mass media invariably focus upon the more pathological elements of youth homelessness and young homeless people. In this way the structural background to youth homelessness is negated, while the problem is frequently portrayed and represented as a personal one, with the result that young homeless people are increasingly being marginalised from mainstream society – a development which simply cannot be congruent with moves towards a 'classless society'.

Let us begin by looking at the recession of the 1980s and the youth unemployment which ensued. If there is any factor that has created the conditions for youth homelessness, it is this recession and the restructuring of the labour market which followed it. After all, it is important to consider the words of David Donnison (1980: 283), who argued that most housing problems are really problems of low income and unemployment.

YOUNG PEOPLE IN THE LABOUR MARKET

The oil crisis in the 1970s heralded an international recession which led to the restructuring of national economies on a global scale. Throughout the Western world, multi-national companies moved manufacturing overseas. Many industries in the UK, such as mining and ship-building, became uneconomic, leaving certain regions without their traditional male jobs – both skilled and unskilled. Large-scale companies, such as British Steel, threw off core workers, cut back on recruitment and subcontracted work on a short-term basis. Many employers, particularly those in the public sector, cut back on workers in response to the recession and to new technologies. Adult unemployment rates rose from 3 per cent in 1961 to 14 per cent in 1988 (Halsey 1988). There is no doubt that monetarist polices of the Conservative Government, with restrictions on public spending and a withdrawal of state intervention, exacerbated unemployment.

Youth unemployment

This recession and the resulting unemployment in the 1980s hit young people disproportionately (Raffe 1987). Unskilled jobs, which had gone to early school-leavers with no qualifications, were the first to go. Apprenticeship schemes were discontinued. Overall, the number of young people going straight from school into employment fell dramatically from 53 per cent in 1976 to 15 per cent in 1986 (Jones and Wallace 1992).

During the late 1980s, the economy picked up with the expansion of the service sector, particularly in the south-east. It was hoped that, when the children of the post-war baby bulge (who reached the labour market in the 1980s) had passed through, the lower number of school-leavers would lessen the pressure on jobs. However, another recession hit the UK in the 1990s, this time affecting the service sector. In 1994/5 the unemployment rate for 18–24-year-olds was around 16 per cent, which is nearly twice the national average, and the gap between general and youth unemployment continues to widen (Evans 1996).

National statistics hide gender, ethnic and regional differences. Throughout this period unemployment rates for young men have been higher than rates for young women. The 1994/5 rate for young men is 18 per cent and for young women 12 per cent. Unemployment is uneven across ethnic groups, with the rate for young black men being 37 per cent. Regionally, rates vary and can be over 50 per cent in certain areas.

Youth training

Youth training schemes were begun in 1983 to replace jobs and to remove 16- and 17-year-olds from the unemployment tables. The element of effective compulsion from 1988 meant that the adjustment of unemployment figures partly achieved its objective, but the inability of many young people to find jobs after schemes meant that this wider aim was not successful. Youth training was widely seen, by both young people and their parents, as an imposition by the Government of 'slave labour' on young people. It was felt that the Government had broken a moral code by not providing jobs for young people (Allatt and Yeandle 1992).

Training allowances (£29–35 a week) have remained relatively constant since 1989 and underlie the current poverty of many young people. It is calculated in 1996 (Evans 1996: 20) that the allowance represents less than a quarter of what a single person would need to spend each week on a 'modest but adequate' budget. The overall poverty of young people has risen, and this is shown by the increase (from a fifth to a third) in their representation in the poorest 10 per cent of households between 1979 and 1993 (Evans 1996: 17). It must be remembered that this statistic covers only young people's households and not young people living at home.

Economic restructuring

This crisis in unemployment was accompanied by a restructuring in the pattern of work (Roberts *et al.* 1985) in which young people were the losers. There was, overall, a decline in regular life-time work, which had been principally for men, and so the recruitment routes into it were closed. Many of the new jobs in the service sector, which was expanding, were taken by married women, who were able to work part-time in a way that young people were not. Moreover, young people are not well positioned to enter self-employment.

Young people also suffered from the effect of the recession on other family members. Labour-market participation became polarised, with many households having either two earners or being entirely dependent on benefit. Research (Payne 1987) showed that young people who were unemployed were more likely to live in households where someone else was unemployed and also to live in poor households (Roll 1990).

When young people do have jobs in the 1990s, these are often low-waged and unstable. The abolition of the Wages Councils, the lack of a minimum wage, chronic unemployment and unsatisfactory training scheme placements have created poorer working conditions for young people than was the case in the 1960s. Studies show that some training schemes simply socialise young people into the low-skilled work, low pay and low positions that they should expect in the 1990s labour market (Bates 1989).

The expansion of education

The expansion of education, particularly further education, must be seen against this loss of work for young people. In the 1960s and before, many young people left school because their families needed their wages. In the 1990s many young people stay on in education because there are no jobs. While the expansion of further education gives opportunities to some, it lengthens young people's period of dependence on their families. Moreover, there are indications that disadvantage is moving up the social spectrum as graduates face unemployment or low-level jobs while the reduction of grants adds part-time jobs and debts to the situation of many students. (Jones and Wallace 1992: 143).

Youth in the labour market and homelessness

The appearance of youth homelessness in the 1980s follows directly the increase in youth unemployment. It was young people particularly who bore the brunt of unemployment in the 1980s, and they continued to lose out in the restructuring of the economy. Youth training and even the expansion of further education did little to create real jobs. Without work and without wages young people cannot access or maintain independent accommodation.

YOUNG PEOPLE IN THE HOUSING MARKET

Increases in youth homelessness are often linked with two related Conservative housing policies – the sharp reduction in 'council' housing and the increase in home-ownership. Let us look at these two policies and then trace their origins in broader changes to the housing market.

The drive for home-ownership and the running down of council housing

From the time that it came to power in 1979, the Conservative Government's drive for home-ownership was pivotal to its housing policy. An important motivation was the hope of gaining votes; the 'right to buy' was a central tenet of an owner-occupying democracy and popular capitalism (Saunders 1990). Between 1979 and 1991 home-ownership grew from 55 per cent to 68 per cent. By 1993, two million council homes had been sold from a stock of 6.5 million in 1979. Capital receipts over the period 1979–93 were £31 billion. As Malpass and Murie (1994) point out, this programme delivered the largest capital receipts of any privatisation programme.

A second reason behind the drive to home-ownership was the

need to cut back on public spending in a recession. However, public spending was not reduced as much as had been expected. Inflation, rising interest rates and house prices raised the cost to the Government of tax-relief and mortgage subsidy. What occurred was a huge transfer in public expenditure away from capital expenditure on housing and subsidies to council housing and towards private household subsidy in the form of Housing Benefit as well as mortgage and tax-relief (Malpass and Murie 1994). The Conservative Government managed this privatisation with little public comment because these changes in subsidy were not easily seen and, more importantly, many voters had individually benefited from the private subsidies.

Both parties build houses

How do these two policies – home-ownership and the run-down of council housing – fit into broader trends in the housing market and the problem of youth homelessness? Malpass and Murie (1994) suggest that, up to 1979, the policies of Right- and Left-wing governments did not vary greatly. From the end of the First World War, the aims of both parties were to build houses – so as to increase living standards, clear slums and compensate for the steady decline of the private rented sector. Production targets and the 'numbers game' were a familiar part of housing politics. It is only in the last decade or so that 'house building targets have ceased to be a measure of ministerial virility' (Malpass and Murie 1994: 65). Although more municipal housing was built under Labour governments, and more privately owned and built housing under the Conservatives, the real divergence in policies came after the late 1960s, at which date the total number of dwellings was broadly equivalent to the number of households.

The decline of the private rented sector

The long-term decline of the private rented sector from the beginning of the century continued irrespective of encouragement of landlords by Conservative governments or control of landlords by Labour. In 1939 private tenants easily outnumbered owner-occupiers and tenants in the public sector. They still formed nearly a quarter of all households in 1966 (Emms 1990). By 1991, however, the private rented sector accounted for less than 8 per cent of the total housing stock. This decline is linked to slum-clearance programmes, increased rent control and comparatively poor rates of return on capital. Young single people, because they are not given priority in council housing, have traditionally had to rely on this declining sector.

The residualisation of council houses

The changing social profile of council tenants constitutes another trend in the housing market. In the first half of the century council housing was of good quality, rents were relatively high, and council-house tenants were relatively well-off. From the 1950s onwards council housing began to change from a tenure for middle-income groups to a tenure of last resort (Forrest and Murie 1988). Changes in rent and the introduction of Housing Benefit made council housing accessible to poorer people who were being cleared from slums or turned out of the declining private rented sector. Wealthier council-house tenants were moving into home-ownership. These factors led to the residualisation of council houses, which became increasingly associated with poverty and management problems.

Increases in single-person households

For young single people, the changing nature of the housing market, and its modification of housing supply, has been significantly compounded in recent years by demographic changes in the popula-tion which have had a dramatic impact upon housing demand – most notably in the rise in the number of single-person households. While the overall population of the UK is ostensibly static, the number of households has been steadily increasing. This is linked with escalating divorce rates, increasing numbers of people of retirement age and a greater tendency to live independently. In 1989 one in four households consisted of just one person, compared with one in twenty in 1911 (Malpass and Murie 1994: 113). These changes increased the pressure on housing but, more significantly, meant a lack of fit between a housing supply built predominately for families and the current demand for single-person accommodation. Interestingly, while the demands by elderly people have been catered for, to a degree at least, demands for social housing by young single people have not been accepted as legitimate by successive Conservative governments.

Increases in homelessness

By the 1970s general homelessness was becoming an issue (Greve *et al.* 1971). Throughout this century, the broader issues of poor housing conditions – homelessness in its broader sense – were addressed through house-building and slum-clearance. Those people more narrowly defined as 'homeless' – those who had been evicted, displaced or were 'roofless' – were often seen as 'undeserving', as against the 'settled' poor of the parish. By the 1960s the numbers of these people were rising because of the decline of the private rented sector, slum-clearance and evictions, particularly following the 1957 Rent Act. The treatment of these homeless people in sex-segregated hostels was highlighted in the film *Cathy Come Home*. Some of these issues were addressed in the 1977 Housing (Homeless Persons) Act, but young single people were largely excluded from the remit of this legislation.

The 1977 Housing (Homeless Persons) Act

Under the 1977 Housing Act, housing departments were given statutory duties to house people who were deemed 'unintentionally homeless', had a local connection and fell into a priority category – of which having dependent children was the most common. At the time of the Act, it was felt that women with children, the elderly and the 'vulnerable' were the categories which would be the least catered for by the private sector, and so they were made the responsibility of the state. The accommodation offered to the priority categories was permanent, because of fears that some Local Authorities would not adequately provide without this safeguard of permanency. Moreover, council houses were in reasonable supply. This Act, however, created a specialism out of homelessness within Housing Departments and housing policy.

In general, single homeless people were not housed under the Act. Young homeless people were not given priority on the basis of their age alone. Whether or not they qualified through 'vulnerability' was open to the interpretation and discretion of the local Housing Department, and most did not. Somerville (1994) tells us that the Joint Charities Group campaigned to give all (including single) homeless people a right to housing, but for the regulations to apply only to those authorities who could cope. The DoE, which dominated the legislation, wanted these statutory rights to be uniform across all authorities, but single people were left out.

Housing and youth homelessness

The claims of young single people to housing have not generally been treated by Conservative governments as legitimate. Until recently, leaving home and gaining housing has been linked with marriage and a family (Leonard 1980). Nevertheless, young people have been affected by these changes in the housing market. The reduction in council housing reduces the overall stock of social housing and increases pressure on an already shrinking private rented sector, and young people are not in a position, in terms of income or life stage, to benefit from the expansion of home-owner-ship. Young people have traditionally depended on the private rented sector when they needed housing, and the overall decline here has affected them. Where young single people have gained council housing today, it is often on hard-to-let estates, which makes successful tenancies less likely. Most significantly, the exclu-sion of young people from the 1977 Housing (Homeless Persons) Act has structured their routes through homelessness and limited the state's response to them. In 1977 youth homelessness was not an issue, but when it became so, in the 1980s, the structures were already set. Proposed changes to the housing legislation in 1996 – whereby 'homeless households' are no longer given priority status, and Local Authorities will not be obliged to offer permanent accommodation – are likely to lead to a downgrading in accommo-dation and services for all.

The nature of the housing market certainly shows a clear discrimination against young people, especially young single people. The gradual reduction of the private rented sector and the more rapid diminution of Local Authority housing stock, coupled with the domination of housing policy and housing tenure by owner occupation, has undoubtedly served to discriminate against all young people seeking to enter the housing market. However, youth homelessness reflects more than simply a general discrimination against young people – an examination of its causes shows that it is specifically the product of cumulative discrimination against those sections of society already experiencing disadvantage. The punitive attacks on the unemployed (especially the unemployed aged under 25) represented by the reduction and withdrawal of benefit can be shown to have had a powerful impact upon the problem of youth homelessness. Similarly, the policy expectation that young people live with and financially rely upon their parents, dependent as it is upon idealised notions of family life, has had a devastating impact upon young people from care or those from homes in which they could not live because of poverty, abuse, conflict or family break-down.

YOUNG PEOPLE AND WELFARE BENEFITS

When the Conservative Government came to power in 1979, Supplementary Benefit payments were making up an increasing amount of the rising social security budget. Those groups who were increasingly claiming were divorced women, single parents, the elderly and unemployed young people. These changes in family structure and rising unemployment had not been predicted in the 1940s by the Beveridge Report. With rising Supplementary Benefit bills, a national recession and an ideological suspicion of 'the nanny state', the Conservative Government cut benefits. These cuts particu-larly targeted young people. It was feared that welfare dependency among the young could spread across a generation. More specifi-cally, it was feared that young people might be encouraged to leave home if their accommodation costs were covered by the state. These cuts were directly aimed at forcing young people back into family homes, where it was assumed that their families could, and should, absorb their living costs.

Benefit changes and youth homelessness

It was only with increasing unemployment that claiming benefit became a major issue for young people. There is, however, little doubt that benefit cuts – particularly in housing costs – were directly responsible for translating youth unemployment into youth homelessness, because they made it more difficult for unemployed young people to access and maintain independent accommodation (Hutson and Liddiard 1991). It is likely that this gap between housing costs and the amount covered by Housing Benefit will be further compounded by new changes to the housing benefit system which came into force in January 1996. Under these changes, a ceiling is placed on the amount of Housing Benefit which is payable to claimants in private rented accommodation. Housing Benefit is restricted on rents which are above the average for the particular type of property in the area, the expectation being that tenants will either negotiate a lower rent or choose cheaper homes – a belief which starkly illustrates the Government's complete ignorance of the realities of the rented sector. In the light of the shortage in housing supply, coupled with the buoyant demand for accommodation, it is difficult to envisage landlords negotiating a lower rent, while cheaper homes are unlikely to be a realistic option for many tenants. In short, the result is likely to be that even more tenants will find themselves simply unable to meet their accommodation costs and will consequently be evicted, with all the attendant problems that this brings. This, and other stricter limits on housing benefits, may have as great an effect on youth homelessness as earlier changes did in 1988.

Let us look briefly at the benefit changes which were introduced in 1988, and which are often taken as a benchmark in accounts of youth homelessness (see Hutson and Liddiard 1994). The most significant change to the benefit system was the 1986 Social Security Act, which actually came into effect in April 1988. One of the main changes that this introduced was the establishment of an age-related – rather than need-related – system of benefit entitlement. Young people under 25 now receive only 80 per cent of the Income Support received by their contemporaries aged 25 or over, while those youngsters aged under 18 who are still eligible for Income Support receive just 60 per cent of those aged over 25 receive – even if they are all in identical circumstances! Indeed, the 1988 Social Security Act saw the end of benefit eligibility for most 16- and 17-year-olds anyway, with only a very small number of exceptions.

Moreover, from this date the calculation of Housing Benefit was modified to exclude elements such as rates and water rates, which were nonetheless still included in rent levels. This was to pave the way for a continuing reduction in Housing Benefit. The discrepancy between real rent levels and Housing Benefit levels then had to be paid out of the claimant's pocket – often out of their diminished Income Support. This discrepancy was greatest in the private rented sector, which was where most young people had to find accommodation. Charges for meals and other services were no longer covered by Housing Benefit. As a result bed and breakfast dropped out as an accommodation option for young people, and those living in hostels had only a few pounds left when these charges were paid.

The rationale behind these changes was to encourage young people under 25 (and particularly under 18) to live with their parents by making it increasingly difficult for them to live independently, at least in terms of finance. Yet, as we shall see, this was simply not an option for many young homeless people.

While these changes to benefits made it increasingly difficult for unemployed young people to pay the rent and maintain their accommodation, the 1986 Social Security Act also made it more difficult for unemployed young people to obtain accommodation in the first place. Before 1988 single payments were available for one-off items such as furniture, a deposit or rent in advance. From April 1988, however, this old system of single payments was replaced with the Social Fund. Under the Social Fund, grants are generally no longer available and instead have been replaced by loans, which are consequently repayable from benefits! However, young homeless people are not a priority group for loans, and in any event deposits to secure rented accommodation are specifically excluded from the Social Fund.

The final blow for young people came with the 1988 Social Security Act, which effectively removed the entitlement of unemployed 16- and 17-year-olds to Income Support. Instead, these young people were expected to be either on a training scheme or dependent on their parents. Claims for hardship payments, which were the main safety-net for this system were, and remain, difficult to obtain and short-term, despite the shortage of training places. The result is that one in seven 16- and 17-year-olds in the workforce (in training, in employment or unemployed) is without an income (Unemployment Unit 1994)! The increase in the proportion of 16/17-year-olds reporting to Centrepoint (from 14 per cent in 1972 to over 50 per cent in 1992) and the increasing numbers of these who have no money at all when they report (75 per cent), reflects the extreme financial difficulties of young people in this age group (Strathdee 1992).

In short, it is possible to claim that the development of a substantial youth homelessness problem in the UK is, in large part, a consequence of the manner in which many young people have been increasingly marginalised by changes in the labour and housing markets, and by the very specific penalisation of unemployed young people, represented by the quite draconian changes to the benefit system witnessed since the late 1980s. In short, far from exemplifying any moves towards a classless society, young people, and particularly young unemployed people, have become increasingly marginalised within mainstream society, the worst manifestation of which has been the dramatic rise in the number of homeless young people.

The situation of young people clearly worsened in the 1980s. Their marginalisation at this time is often compared with their situation in the 1960s. Let us look at this more carefully. There is no doubt that the key to the position of young people at that time were the plentiful jobs for unskilled school-leavers. Moreover, wages were near to adult rates. Young people were able to change jobs, often to improve their situation. This was a time when the general population had 'never had it so good' and young people, with jobs and without family responsibilities, 'had money in their pockets'. It was this wealth which financed the expansion of working-class youth leisure and youth cultures.

The wage was the 'golden key' to adulthood at that time (Willis 1984). It was the wage, or more specifically the wage of the male breadwinner, that enabled young people to get married. It was generally only on marriage that young people left home, and marriage was a main route into housing (Leonard 1980). Accommodation for single young people was not generally an issue, nor was claiming benefit at a time of full employment. Jones and Wallace (1992) suggest that this connection between getting a job, getting married and having children only coincided in the 1960s; both before and afterwards the fit was less neat. Moreover, it is likely that before this time pay for young people was low, as each cohort of school-leavers was replaced by younger, cheaper youngsters.

This suggests that young people lost ground in the 1980s in relation to a relatively recent and short-lived affluence and independence during the 1960s and 1970s. It represents a massive deterioration in the situation of young people not paralleled by any other group in society, let alone such a broad one. One can speculate that it was able to happen because of the political weakness of young people, who seek their individual independence rather than political rights, and because of the willingness of so many families to take up the strain. There is no doubt that the family, and family support, is an important part of this development. After all, the expectation behind the restrictions on welfare benefits for young unemployed people was that these youngsters would instead become increasingly reliant upon their parents and family – an expectation which was wholly misplaced in the context of young homeless people, many of whom are simply estranged from their families.

YOUNG PEOPLE AND THE FAMILY

Several studies have looked at the way in which working-class families did support their young people when youth unemployment struck in the 1980s. Parents housed young unemployed people and, where they could, compensated for the lack of a wage. There are detailed accounts of mothers giving young people money so that they could go out and socialise and 'have money in their pockets', as was the then expectation for young single people (Hutson and Jenkins 1989). However, this support was not straightforward. Through such support, parents tried to maintain central social values, such as the work ethic. They had fears that, if young people were to get used to being on the dole, they might never want proper work. There was a tension between the two strands of parenting – the love and comfort, versus the need to urge young people to get up in the morning, work and eventually to 'settle down' (Allatt and Yeandle 1992). Other studies showed that families cannot cope indefinitely with the strains of the 'dole' (Coffield *et al.* 1986; Wallace 1987). As unemployment, longer education and later marriage all make young people increasingly dependent, families cannot go on supporting them, 'as if the household budget was a bottomless pit' (Jones and Wallace 1992: 78). Young people began to leave home, seek accommodation and have children without a regular wage.

While many young people can rely on family support, others cannot. From the late 1980s it was noted that a high proportion (⅓–½) of young people using homelessness services had a background in care (O'Mahony 1988; Randall 1988; Hutson and Liddiard 1991). Moreover, those young people who became homeless after leaving home generally had no choice but to go, because of family conflict, and emotional, physical or sexual abuse (Hendessi 1992; Hutson and Liddiard 1994), and they were leaving home early, at the age of 16 or younger. For such young people, family support has broken down. It was being made plain to the Government by a plethora of agencies, researchers and academics (see O'Mahony 1988; Randall 1988; Hutson and Liddiard 1991; Hendessi 1992; Hutson and Liddiard 1994) that the majority of homeless young people could not return to or rely on their families for support, and that housing and benefit policies based on this assumption were putting the nation's most vulnerable young people seriously at risk. However, we would argue that the response to this profile of youth homelessness – from government and others – has simply further marginalised young homeless people.

THE RESPONSE TO YOUTH HOMELESSNESS

Voluntary agencies

As research was showing that young homeless people were vulnerable and not able to return to their families, children's charities were also campaigning for them. Since these young people fell outside the remit of social service departments, because of their age, and generally outside the responsibility of housing departments, it was the voluntary sector which provided the majority of services for them. Specific organisations were set up in the 1970s, such as Centrepoint, Alone in London and the Soho Project. In the 1980s the major children's charities – Barnardos, National Children's Homes, the Children's Society – moved into the field of youth homelessness. In many cases resources and workers were switched from residential children's care (children's homes were being closed at that time, because residential care was no longer seen as appropriate for many children). Resources were transferred into what was seen as a new problem – youth homelessness.

Statutory responsibilities

The concern of these bodies and of the Government lay behind Part III of the Children Act 1989, implemented in 1991. This Act brought these vulnerable young people under statutory responsibility. This responsibility lay with the local authorities as a whole, but social services were the lead agency. Local Authorities were expected to plan and provide services for these young people, including accommodation. Support was expected to come from social services, in partnership with the voluntary sector, and housing was expected to come from Housing Departments, in partnership with Housing Associations.

Questions of definition hindered the necessary co-operation between social services and Housing Departments. While the latter operate to the definition of 'vulnerability' under the Housing Acts

1977/85, social services are bound by the 'children-in-need' definition. These are not the same. Joint work was also difficult because
of a lack of resources. For example, a survey by CHAR in 1993
found that only 62 per cent of social services departments surveyed
stated that they accepted homeless 16- and 17-year-olds as children
in need (CHAR 1993). Moreover a let-out clause in the Children
Act states that a housing authority must respond to requests from
social services only if the request 'is compatible with its own statutory duties and obligations and does not unduly prejudice the
discharge of its functions'.

There is no doubt that the Children Act led to an increased
awareness by Local Authorities of the problems of homeless young
people. In many areas, after-care teams were set up within social
services, and housing and support schemes for young people were
also set up (Hutson 1995). However, this tended to happen only in
urban areas – where voluntary agencies were already active and
where some adolescent specialism existed within social services
prior to the Act. More importantly, services have centred on a
narrow category of young people – care-leavers – rather than
including other homeless young people who have not left care. If
these latter young people are assessed at all, they may get advice but
not services. Moreover, very few services go to young people over
18. This reflects social services' priorities in a situation where there
is an acute lack of resources.

Thus, although statutory responsibilities were acknowledged
through the Children Act, a lack of resources led to restrictive definitions. One group of young people – care-leavers – have acquired a
degree of 'special needs' status, and they may be excluded from the
further restrictions proposed by the Conservative Government to
housing legislation and housing benefits. However, many disadvantaged young people are left out. Moreover, as fewer children are
taken into care in the first place, fewer young people will qualify for
any kind of special status. Thus, while the Children Act acknowledged the extreme vulnerability of those young people who are
unable to live at home and gave a potential for statutory responsibility, trends in youth unemployment, restricted benefits, cuts in
public spending and a lack of social housing work against the
implementation of the Act at all levels.

The Children Act has been the only attempt to deal with youth
homelessness through specific legislation. Responses to youth
homelessness, both before and after this Act, have been in terms of

'special' housing and accommodation projects. Usually such projects offer young people temporary housing and teach independent living skills for one to two years, and where possible move-on accommodation is found. Many of these projects are set up by voluntary agencies but sometimes with government funding. While the impact of these projects on local-level provision and on good practice should not be forgotten (Hutson 1993), they cannot have a wide or general influence, as they do not alter the housing or employment situation for many young people, which is ultimately the key to resolving the problem of youth homelessness. Moreover, the operation of these projects can come under threat from broader policies – such as housing policies and benefit restrictions.

This setting up of special projects, rather than working on a broader policy level, is common throughout Europe. The UK is one of only two EC countries not to have a minister who is responsible, in some way, for youth issues (House of Lords 1991). Through the emphasis on family conflict and the narrowing of the client group outlined above, youth homelessness has become a 'social problem' rather than an economic issue. This type of response to 'social problems', by philanthropy and special projects, is embedded in political practice and social values throughout the Western world. In this way even the policy responses to youth homelessness have served to marginalise these young people further. Indeed, this process of marginalisation is compounded by the nature of much research into youth homelessness.

RESEARCH AND YOUTH HOMELESSNESS

While earlier research into youth homelessness stressed structural factors (O'Mahony 1988; Hutson and Liddiard 1991), there has recently been more of an emphasis upon the family problems of young people, problems which go back into childhood. This emphasis is evident in many studies from the USA, where the term 'street children', rather than young homeless people, is used (Robertson 1990). In a study of young homeless people in London and Sydney, Downing-Orr (1994) also suggests that the majority of the homeless youngsters come from families which are dysfunctional or problematic in some way, and that they leave directly because of serious conflict. She indicates that this youth–parental alienation begins in early to middle childhood. Moreover, these young people feel betrayed by childhood institutions, such as school or care, and so do not turn to them for support. Similarly, a recent study (Centrepoint 1996), of young runaways (14–16 years) reporting to a safe house in London, shows that many come from dysfunctional families. The young people's accounts suggest that conflicts arose not from their parents' concern for them but from what they felt to be lack of care or hate. These young people felt that their parents had negative feelings towards them, and some felt singled out among their siblings in this. In many cases these feelings go back into middle childhood. These young people were distrustful of adults and tended to be unattached from school or other forms of peer or adult support.

There are several explanations for this current change in emphasis from structural explanations of youth homelessness to explanations of family pathology. On the one hand it may reflect an acceptance, on the part of researchers and campaigners, of economic trends such as the disappearance of work for early school-leavers. It may also reflect the failure of research findings to bring a change in Government policies. Explanations and solutions also have an inexorable tendency to be continually changed. In this way, governments, campaigning bodies and agencies can appear to be achieving progress while little in the outside structures is altering. Whatever the reasons for this notable change in emphasis, the high-lighting of family pathology as a significant contributing factor in youth homelessness has served to further marginalise young home-less people as being somehow different and distinct from mainstream society. This is undoubtedly compounded by the treat-ment that youth homelessness receives at the hands of the mass media.

THE MASS MEDIA AND YOUTH HOMELESSNESS

In representing homelessness, the press concentrates on street homelessness, because of the stark contrasts it gives, together with its connection with prostitution, drugs, drink and death (Hutson and Liddiard 1994; Liddiard 1996). The public nature of street homelessness also makes it easy to film. The mass media also draws upon street scenes and often uses the drama documentary to depict young people's careers on the street. In this way, youth homelessness is presented as a social problem somehow distinct and separate from the mainstream housing and labour-market issues which lie at its heart. The particular way in which youth homelessness is presented can be seen by contrasting it with the issue of mortgage repossession, which, although a cause of homelessness, is featured less often in the press and media. It is not presented with photographs or drama documentaries but is usually an item with other economic issues. Youth homelessness is thus treated as a narrow social problem by the press and media reporting, and in this way the young homeless themselves become further marginalised as somehow distinct. Importantly, this marginalisation is not distinct or separate from that which occurs in terms of policy responses. On the contrary, there is often a close relationship between the two – for instance, the Government is well aware of these press images and considerable efforts have been put into clearing homeless people off the streets.

The marginalisation of young people in general, and young home-less people specifically, is thus evident in a variety of different contexts – in terms of broad changes to the labour and housing markets; in terms of quite specific attacks upon unemployed young people through draconian changes to the benefit regime; in terms of policy responses to the problem of youth homelessness; and even in terms of the media representations of homeless young people. The process by which such a large and significant proportion of society has been effectively excluded from mainstream society and marginalised is hardly synonymous with the notion of a 'classless society'. On the contrary, these processes have undoubtedly served to produce an increasingly divided and iniquitous society. Indeed, this is made more pronounced by the fact that young homeless people are disproportionately represented among the lower social classes.

Interestingly, the connection between youth homelessness and class has been assumed rather than examined. We know that young people who become homeless are more likely to come from house-holds where parents are on benefit (Jones 1993). We know that many young homeless people come from care, and that young people from poorer families are more likely to end up in care (Bebbington and Miles 1989). It is likely that – as young people become more dependent on, and expensive for, their families, because of unemployment and low benefits – those from the poorest homes may be pushed out, or, once they have left, stay away (Hutson *et al.* 1995). We can assume 'when the state takes away the safety net of social citizenship, that some families can step in and provide financial assistance, food and housing whilst others cannot' (Jones and Wallace 1992: 116).

However, there is a lack of data to support this assumed link between poverty, social class and homelessness. One reason is that, while surveys have generally been aware of gender and ethnicity as variables to be monitored, the social-class background of young people has not been asked for. It is felt to be intrusive to inquire about the occupation of parent(s), particularly at agencies where young people are treated as independent people. There is another reason why the class link with youth homelessness has not been stressed. This is because of the need, by campaigning agencies and charities, to stress the universal nature of the problem. If homelessness can affect 'the boy/girl down the road', then the public and the politician can be drawn in to identify with the problems and the risks (Liddiard and Hutson 1991; Hutson and Liddiard 1994).

However, the link with homelessness and conflict between parent(s) and young people has already been stressed. Such conflict is not restricted to poor families. Moreover, many poor families support their children even when this entails considerable sacrifice, as we saw with the working-class families supporting unemployed children (Hutson and Jenkins 1989). If divorce and step-parent families are connected with increased rates of homelessness, then these occur across classes. The marginalisation of youth within social policy, which has been stressed in this chapter, cuts across class and this can now be seen in the worsening financial situation of students, even in higher education (Ford et al. 1994).

THE FUTURE?

This chapter has focused in some detail upon the processes by which young people in general, and unemployed and homeless young people more specifically, have been increasingly marginalised from mainstream society in recent years. However, what of the future? With the rhetoric of the 'classless society', are we likely to witness growing moves towards the full inclusion of young people, and particularly young homeless people, into contemporary society? The short and somewhat depressing answer is – no.

On the one hand, the peripheral position of young people in the labour and housing markets has now become well established, while the vulnerability of national labour markets to international and global economic developments means that, to some degree at least, these issues may be beyond the control of national governments. However, even when there is clear and unequivocal evidence that

Government policies are directly contributing to a rise in the number of homeless young people – as there is in relation to the benefit restrictions imposed on young people in 1988 – there has been complete inaction on the part of government. On the contrary, we are now witnessing even further restrictions in welfare entitlements. One can only conclude from such inaction that John Major's allusions to a 'classless society' amount to nothing more than empty rhetoric.

However, what of the future? With the election of a new Labour Government at the recent General Election, what are the potential prospects for young people in general and young homeless people in particular? What policy statements there have been from New Labour show much in terms of presentation, but frustratingly little in terms of concrete commitment. Indeed, some of the statements from Labour seem to suggest that they may have even less appreciation of the problems facing young unemployed and homeless people than the current government. There have certainly been some quite contradictory statements coming from New Labour in relation to its housing policies. For example, Labour policy statements have committed themselves to a release of some £6 billion worth of capital receipts from the sale of council housing for new house-building, while simultaneously claiming that a future Labour government would not increase the PSBR (the Public Sector Borrowing Requirement). Yet, as a number of commentators have pointed out, there is a close relationship between capital receipts and the PSBR, so that releasing capital receipts would increase the PSBR (Birch 1996). There thus appear to be a number of unanswered questions in relation to Labour's housing policy, while the party simultaneously appear to have few qualms about adopting wholesale the current government's marginalisation of young people, and particularly young unemployed people, for crude political objectives. In short, the prospects for young homeless people in particular, and young homeless people more generally, appear to be bleak.

CONCLUSIONS

Youth homelessness is often linked with specific Conservative policies, such as the 1988 Social Security Act, which saw 16- and 17-year-olds lose their entitlement to Income Support. Certainly, there is no doubt whatsoever that such policies have played a highly influential role in inflating the scale of youth homelessness in the UK, and we have argued elsewhere that simply re-examining these benefit restrictions will make an important difference to alleviating the problem of youth homelessness (Hutson and Liddiard 1994). However, we have also suggested that if these issues are set against broader trends in the housing market, and particularly the labour market – which can be highly dependent upon international and even global economic developments – then the factors behind the disadvantages of many young people are unlikely to alter quickly with a change of government.

This chapter highlights the way in which young people have been marginalised. This marginalisation is not new, although it clearly has become more pronounced. Even before the cutbacks in the 1980s, for instance, young single people's access to independent welfare payments and housing was tenuous. The deterioration in the situation of young people and the increases in homelessness in the 1980s followed a period of full employment and relative affluence for young people in the 1960s, which was a relatively short-lived phase. The marginalisation of young people, particularly that of young unemployed people which was evident in the changes to benefit entitlement, has rested heavily upon the assumption that young people can be looked after by their families. Where this is not possible – when young people have been in care or where there is conflict in the family – then homelessness has occurred.

Because of general economic trends and the marginalisation of young people within them, many young people are disadvantaged. Youth homelessness has symbolised this disadvantage and has been taken up particularly by the press and the media. There is a danger, however, that in focusing on youth homelessness, attention will be focused only on the extremity. Even within youth homelessness, the response has been to a narrower client group. Services from the Children Act are often restricted to a small and diminishing group of young people – care-leavers. The Government has funded special projects to provide services in certain localities, rather than developing youth policies. Current research has moved away from the examination of structural causes to looking at dysfunctional families. The press features life on the streets rather than the many more young people sleeping on floors or moving between insecure accommodation.

It is important that the general marginalisation of young people, particularly unemployed and homeless young people, and the structural reasons behind it – the labour market, the housing market and the welfare system – are put back on general political agendas with youth in mind. Until they are, it is difficult to see how the profound inequities and discrimination against young people that the past seventeen years have witnessed, which has its most disturbing manifestation in terms of youth homelessness, can possibly be addressed.

REFERENCES

Allatt, P. and Yeandle, S. (1992) *Youth Unemployment and the Family: Voices of Disordered Times*, London: Routledge.

Bates, I. (1989) *No Bleeding, Whining Minnies: The Role of YTS in Class and Gender Reproduction*, ESRC 16–19 Occasional Paper 23, London: SSRU, City University.

Bebbington, A. and Miles, J. (1989) 'The background of children who enter Local Authority care', *British Journal of Social Work* 19(5): 349–68.

Birch, J. (1996) 'The Midas touch', *Roof*, January/February: 24–7

Centrepoint (1996) *Nowhere to Hide: Giving Young Runaways a Voice*, London: Centrepoint.

CHAR (1993) *Plans No Action: Summary of Findings of Preliminary Research into the Children Act and Homeless Young People*, London: CHAR

Coffield, F., Borrill, C. and Marshall, S. (1986) *Growing Up at the Margins*, Milton Keynes: Open University Press.

Donnison, D. (1980) 'A policy for housing', *New Society*, 54(938): 283–4.

Downing-Orr, K. (1994) *Alienation During Childhood and the Process of Becoming Homeless*, unpublished D.Phil. thesis, University of Oxford.

Emms, P. (1990) *Social Housing: A European Dilemma*, Bristol: University of Bristol.

Evans, A. (1996) *People Don't Choose to be Homeless*, Report of the National Inquiry into the Prevention of Homelessness amongst Young People, London: CHAR.

Ford, J., Bosworth, D. and Wilson, R. (1994) *Part-time Work and Full-time Higher Education* ESRC End of Term Report, Swindon, ESRC.

Forrest, R. and Murie, A. (1988) *Selling the Welfare State*, London: Routledge.

Greve, J., Page, D. and Greve, S. (1971) *Homelessness in London*, London: Scottish Academic Press.

Halsey, A. (ed.) (1988) *British Social Trends since 1900: A Guide to the Changing Social Structure of Britain*, London: Macmillan.

Hendessi, M. (1992) *4 in 10: Report on Young Women Who Become Homeless as a Result of Sexual Abuse*, London: CHAR.

House of Lords Select Committee on the European Communities (1991) *Young People in the European Communities*, London: HMSO.

Hutson, S. (1993) *Accommodation and Support for Young People: A Survey of Projects*, Cardiff: Welsh Office.

—— (1995) *Care-leavers and Young Homeless People in Wales: The Exchange of Good Practice*, Cardiff: The Welsh Office.

Hutson, S. and Jenkins, R. (1989) *Taking the Strain: Families, Unemployment and the Transition to Adulthood*, Milton Keynes: Open University Press.

Hutson, S. and Liddiard, M. (1991) *Young and Homeless in Wales: Government Policies, Insecure Accommodation and Agency Support*, Swansea: University of Wales.

—— (1994) *Youth Homelessness: The Construction of a Social Issue*, London: Macmillan.

Hutson, S., Sutton, M. and Thomas, J. (1995) *The Housing and Support Needs of Young Homeless People in Merthyr Tydfil*, Occasional Paper No. 28, Swansea: University of Wales.

Jones, G. (1993) *Regulated Entry into the Housing Market? The Process of Leaving Home*, Working Paper 2, Edinburgh: Centre for Educational Sociology.

Jones, G. and Wallace, C. (1992) *Youth, Family and Citizenship*, Buckingham: Open University Press.

Leonard, D. (1980) *Sex and Generation: A Study of Courtship and Weddings*, London: Tavistock.

Liddiard, M. (1996) *Homelessness: The Media, Public Attitudes and Policy Making*, unpublished paper given at Social Policy Association Annual Conference, Sheffield Hallam University.

Liddiard, M. and Hutson, S. (1991) 'Homeless young people and runaways – agency definitions and processes', *Journal of Social Policy* 20(3): 365–88.

Malpass, P. and Murie, A. (1994) *Housing Policy and Practice* (4th ed.), London: Macmillan.

O'Mahony, B. (1988) *A Capital Offence: The Plight of the Young Single Homeless in London*, London: Routledge.

Payne, J. (1987) 'Does unemployment run in families?', *Sociology* 21(2): 199–214.

Raffe, D. (1987) 'Youth unemployment in the United Kingdom 1979–1984', in P. Brown and D. Ashton (eds) *Education and Youth Labour Markets*, Lewes: Falmer Press.

Randall, G. (1988) *No Way Home: Homeless Young People in Central London*, London: Centrepoint.

Roberts, B., Finnegan, R. and Gallie, D. (eds) (1985) *New Approaches to Economic Life*, Manchester: Manchester University Press.

Robertson, M. (1990) 'Characteristics and Circumstances of Homeless Adolescence in Hollywood', unpublished paper presented at the American Psychological Association, Boston.

Roll, J. (1990) *Young people: Growing up in the Welfare State*, Occasional Paper No. 10, London: Family Policy Studies Centre.

Saunders, P. (1990) *A Nation of Home Owners*, London: Unwin Hyman.

Somerville, P. (1994) 'Homelessness policy in Britain', *Policy and Politics*, 22(3): 163–78.

Strathdee, R. (1992) *No Way Back: Homeless Sixteen and Seventeen Year Olds in the 90s*, London: Centrepoint.

Unemployment Unit (1994) *Working Brief*, Issue 52, London: Unemployment Unit.

Wallace, C. (1987) *For Richer, For Poorer: Growing Up in and out of Work*, London: Tavistock Publications.

Willis, P. (1984) 'Youth unemployment', *New Society*, 67 (1114).

Chapter 7

Youth crime, social change and crime control in Britain and France in the 1980s and 1990s

John Pitts

INTRODUCTION

The economic changes which occurred in Europe during the administrations of Margaret Thatcher and John Major, and the redistribution of wealth, opportunity and political power that these governments fostered, have transformed the class structure of contemporary Britain. Far from promoting classlessness, they have deepened class divisions and exacerbated the effects of economic globalisation upon the most vulnerable. These developments have also precipitated profound changes in the nature and distribution of youth crime. In this chapter I shall consider the ways in which two governments, those of Britain and France, defined and responded to these changing class relations and the changing forms of youth crime and social disorder they spawned in the 1980s and 1990s. In doing so, I shall draw upon recent research undertaken in two established 'working-class' neighbourhoods – one in London and one in Paris. In conclusion, I shall explore the implications of these findings for a future British government concerned to make an intelligent response to the problems of social cohesion and social order generated by the radical changes in class relations identified in this chapter.

THE RISING CRIME RATE

Between 1981 and 1991 the number of crimes recorded in the UK rose from around 3.5 million per annum to almost six million. Government ministers were temporarily heartened in 1988, when recorded crime dropped by 5 per cent, and for a time it seemed that their investment in law and order, a real increase of 87 per cent during the Conservatives' period in office, was at last paying off. But recorded crime rose sharply again from the end of 1989, climbing by 17 per cent in 1990 and a further 16 per cent in 1991. Although the numbers of young people aged between 10 and 17 in the population of England and Wales fell by around 25 per cent during the 1980s, and the decade also saw a dramatic reduction in prosecutions of children aged 10 to 14, recorded crime committed by juveniles rose by 54 per cent (Hagell and Newburn 1994). Alongside this, the British Crime Survey revealed that we were not only witnessing an increase in the volume of crime, but significant changes in its nature and geographical distribution as well (Hope 1994). To understand this changing pattern of crime we need to return to the economic and social changes which occurred in Britain during the 1980s and 1990s.

The redistribution of work and wealth

The economic recession of the early 1980s triggered a sharp rise in unemployment in general and youth unemployment in particular. In the longer term, the progressive de-industrialisation of the British economy led to the erosion of higher-paid, permanent, skilled and semi-skilled jobs in the manufacturing sector. As the 1980s progressed it became evident that youth unemployment was now structural and permanent, rather than cyclical and temporary. Moreover, because this new form of unemployment was, in part, a product of technological change, it was largely unresponsive to economic growth. In 1986, in an effort to strengthen the resolve of the young unemployed, the government withdrew the social security benefits of 15- to 18-year-olds, directing them instead to a 'guaranteed place' on a training scheme. However, few of these training places materialised. Meanwhile, changes in the tax and benefits systems meant that between 1981 and 1991 the number of workers earning half the national average wage or less – the Council of Europe poverty line – rose from 900,000 to 2,400,000. In the same period those earning over twice the national average rose from 1,800,000 to 3,100,000.

Housing the 'have-nots'

Economic restructuring, youth unemployment, the redistribution of wealth in favour of the already prosperous and benefit reductions were necessary components, but it was the introduction of market mechanisms into the management of public-sector housing by the Thatcher administration which gave the final impetus to the radical transformation of crime and victimisation on the poorest council estates in Britain in the 1980s (Hope 1994). As the decade progressed, relatively prosperous elderly and higher-income families left these estates in the inner cities or on their peripheries, to be replaced by poorer, younger, often lone-parent, families (Page 1993). At the beginning of the 1980s the average household income of council-house residents was 73 per cent of the national average; at the beginning of the 1990s this had fallen to 48 per cent. By 1995 over 50 per cent of council households had no breadwinner (Rowntree Foundation 1996). The estates which experienced the greatest changes saw increasing concentrations of children, teenagers, young single adults and the single elderly. Poor, young Black and Asian families constituted a significant segment of this population in some regions. These neighbourhoods also became a last resort for residents who had previously been homeless, hospitalised or imprisoned, and for refugees from political persecution.

As a result, those people most vulnerable to criminal victimisation and those most likely to victimise them were progressively thrown together on the poorest housing estates in Britain. Rated on a ten-point scale, by 1991 residents in the highest-crime neighbourhoods experienced twice as much property crime and four times as much personal crime as residents in the next-worst category. In their study of one such estate, Hope and Foster (1992) discovered a five-fold increase in burglaries over a three-year period.

Neighbourhood destabilisation

One of the first casualties of these changes was a sense of common purpose. As Tim Hope (1995) suggests, some sense of connectedness or common identity, however slight, is crucial if the social and economic well-being of residents is to be defended, since it is the basis for a 'virtuous circle' of mutually reinforcing neighbourhood factors which determine both the quality of life and the standard of living in poor neighbourhoods (McGahey 1986). These factors include demographic stability, the availability of appropriate housing, the quality and strength of schools, social services and family support. These factors are also the precondition for the effective exercise of informal social control within neighbourhoods.

However, these factors are in no small part a product of the level of participation in neighbourhood social and political organisations, which is in turn a product of the quality of interpersonal and inter-group relationships in the neighbourhood. Participation in social and political organisations enhances a neighbourhood's capacity to exert control over crime and victimisation. Such 'horizontal integration' – people getting together to identify shared concerns – is a precondition for greater vertical integration: in which neighbourhood representatives make relationships with, and act as advocates for, the neighbourhood in order to extract resources from those political groupings, state bureaucracies and social agencies with formal responsibility for the problem of crime. It is not that these 'social' factors are more important than economic forces in shaping the destinies of neighbourhoods, rather that they are in themselves an economic factor, and a precondition for the closer integration of a neighbourhood with its economic environment.

Neighbourhood destabilisation erodes both formal and informal economic links. In the 1980s and 1990s young people in high-crime neighbourhoods have become progressively isolated from formal opportunities in the economic mainstream, while informal access to work, based on personal relationships with older working people in the same neighbourhood, has evaporated (Wilson 1987). Their predicament has been compounded by the wide-scale evacuation of inner-city retail, industrial and commercial firms to the new shopping centres and business and industrial parks on the periphery. Paradoxically, as a result of recent policy changes, this exodus has also seen the departure of governmental training resources, which now follow businesses rather than those seeking work.

Market society and the depoliticisation of the public domain

In the 1980s cutbacks in local-government expenditure resulted in the withdrawal of many of the youth-service, community-development and social-welfare services which had previously contributed to the quality of communal life and social cohesion in socially deprived neighbourhoods. However, it is not simply that there was greater need and fewer organisations and individuals available to respond to that need. In the 1980s the nature of both public services and 'publics' themselves has changed. The 1980s witnessed a substantial redistribution of political power from local to central government and the parallel introduction of the 'market forces' into public services (Hutton 1995). This introduction of the quasi-market has spawned new 'slim-line', 'customer-oriented', 'managerially-driven' public services, attuned to the 'effective demand' of individual customers or, more usually, institutional 'purchasers' acquiring services on their behalf. Structurally disconnected from, and therefore unresponsive to, local publics, local politics and local problems, public services were increasingly directed by bureaucratically determined 'targets', shaped in accordance with self-referential performance indicators imposed by central government (Clarke *et al.* 1994; Le Grand 1996). As such, public services were no longer a medium whereby private troubles could be translated into public issues (Mills 1957). Elliot Currie (1991) argues that the advent of 'market society' has been a major factor in the erosion of the capacity of citizens in multiply deprived neighbourhoods to cope with problems amongst young people.

The youth crime implosion

The crime and violence in these neighbourhoods is implosive in that it is committed by, and against, local residents. This intra-neighbourhood crime pattern is a distinguishing characteristic of high-crime areas in Britain (Forrester *et al.* 1988; Hope 1995). Their other distinguishing feature is that the young people involved in this crime appear not to grow out of it (Graham and Bowling 1995). Hagan (1993) has observed that pre-eminent among the factors which make for higher levels of crime in these neighbourhoods is that young people who, under other circumstances, would have grown out of crime, leaving it behind with other adolescent enthusiasms, become more deeply and more seriously embedded in a criminal way of life. This, in turn, means that the composition of adolescent peer groups is older, and so, for example, links may be forged between criminal neophytes of 14 and old stagers of 25 (Pitts 1995; Hope 1995). Thus conflicts which begin in the school quickly spill over into the neighbourhood, while the school increasingly becomes a forum for the enactment of neighbourhood conflict.

YOUTH JUSTICE IN THE 1980s AND 1990s

Although, as we have seen, the government's economic and social policies have had a profound effect on the nature and distribution of crime in Britain in the 1980s and 1990s, the erratic twists and turns in the politics, policy and practice of youth justice since 1979 have had little or nothing to do with the changing shape of youth crime. They are better understood as a product of the government's attempts to manage the tensions between its political ideology, economic reality and the desire to be re-elected. This has meant that the issue of youth crime has sometimes occupied the centre of the political stage, most notably in the early 1980s and the early 1990s, while at others it has been pushed out of the political limelight and placed in the hands of the 'experts'.

1979–1982: The restoration of the rule of law

For some time, Margaret Thatcher's first term in office looked as if it might also be her last. The economic recession deepened and unemployment soared, giving the lie to promises of new freedoms and greater prosperity. Faced with this situation, the Government attempted to deflect public attention from the economy to crime and, in doing so, to present itself as the only party with the moral and political grit to 'win the war' against it.

At the heart of Conservative criminal justice rhetoric between 1979 and 1982 was the commitment to the restoration of 'the rule of the law' and the pledge to render the streets of Britain safe once more for law-abiding citizens (Hall S. *et al.* 1978; Lea and Young 1984; Pitts 1996). The 1982 Criminal Justice Act (CJA) was heralded as the law which, by restoring the powers of the police and the bench, would make good Mrs Thatcher's 'law and order' promises. Yet, behind the scenes, it was clear that the youth justice system inherited by the Thatcher government was a mess; an incoherent mixture of welfare-oriented measures introduced by the Children and Young Persons Act (1969) and the Attendance Centres, Detention Centres and Borstals of a previous era. It was a system which was locking up more and more less problematic children and young people. This was forcing older juveniles up into the adult system, where they were placing enormous strains on a prison system which was itself at bursting point. Moreover, youth justice was one of the many areas of government spending perceived to be spiralling out of control, and this was acutely embarrassing for an administration committed to 'small government' and 'good house-keeping' (Scull 1977).

1982–1992: The fiscal crisis and decarceration

Having been saved from electoral defeat by the Falklands War, the second Thatcher administration, now in the thrall of monetarism, confronted the reality of Britain's fiscal crisis (Scull 1977). The crisis centred upon the inability of the state to maintain existing welfare and crime-control services in the face of rising costs, competing demands on state expenditure, largely from unemployment benefit, mounting political pressure to reduce taxation and a significant reduction in the tax-paying population. As a result, the period between 1982 and 1992 witnessed a sustained attempt to contain the burgeoning costs of crime control and the penal system. This led to the development, by Home Secretaries Brittan, Hurd, Waddington and Baker, of a highly pragmatic strategy of 'delinquency management' rooted in a profound scepticism about the efficacy of imprisonment or the possibility of rehabilitation outside it. Thus, the 1982 CJA, its blood-curdling rhetoric notwithstanding, was the law which initiated the rationalisation of the youth justice system in England and Wales.

An uneasy alliance

In 1983 the DHSS launched the Intermediate Treatment Initiative, in which £15,000,000 was committed to the provision of 4,500 alternatives to custody over the following three years. The Initiative required an uneasy alliance, between the youth justice lobby – comprising youth justice professionals, penal reform groups, progressive Home Office civil servants and academics – and a neo-conservative 'law and order' government, which yielded some remarkable results. Between 1981 and 1989 the numbers of juveniles imprisoned in Young Offenders Institutions fell from 7,700 to 1,900 per annum.

The Initiative succeeded because the desire of the youth justice lobby to limit the state's intervention in the lives of children and young people in trouble articulated with the government's cost-cutting imperatives and its commitment to 'small government'. Besides, for the neo-conservatives, who were gaining increasing influence within government, the state had no mandate to intervene in the social causes of crime. If the problem was to be solved at all, it would be solved by punishing serious criminals harshly and sending those on the threshold of crime an unequivocal message about the consequences of their actions. In Britain, before 1992, ministers chose to send these unequivocal messages to young offenders in community-based alternatives to custody. Many members of the Conservative government were aware that the social changes wrought by neo-conservative economic policy probably fostered youth crime but, such was the power of neo-conservative ideology in the mid-1980s, there was a tacit acceptance that this was a price worth paying. In consequence the government opted for the manipulation of the apparatus of justice and crime control and the media rather than social intervention in high-crime neighbourhoods.

Political dissonance

There was, of course, a considerable ideological distance between the pessimistic, and apparently quiescent, governmental stance on youth crime in Britain in the 1980s and that of the traditionally punitive rank and file of the Conservative Party. The bridge was provided by the 'justice model', which began life in the 1970s as a strategic alternative to traditional forms of social-work intervention with young people in trouble (Thorpe *et al.* 1980). The justice model was sold to the key political, professional and media constituencies as a tough, confrontational, non-custodial response to 'high-tariff' offenders, the scientific validity of which was vouchsafed by cognitive psychology. The justice model accorded closely with both the administrative and political imperatives of contemporary government criminal justice strategy. The administrative fit was achieved by an individualised of mode of correctional 'treatment', the timing of which was endlessly elastic, determined by the length of the community-based penalty imposed upon the 'young offender'. The political fit was vouchsafed by the treatment's obvious remoralising objectives and its claims to effect sustainable behavioural change.

It is at least doubtful that either the youth justice lobby or Home Office ministers actually believed that the justice model 'worked'. Thus their involvement in the manipulation of ideas and the reproduction of correctional practices was essentially pragmatic. Both sides chose to live in this state of 'bad faith' because the alliance they had entered was working so well for both parties that to 'rock the boat' by revealing the fiction which underlay the endeavour would have been strategic suicide.

The new penology

It was this collusive silence which facilitated the annexation of the youth justice lobby's radical minimalism by an emergent 'new penology' which was the central achievement of Home Office criminal justice strategy in the 1980s (Feely and Simon 1992). The technology of the new penology, as it developed in Britain, consisted of *risk of custody scales*, which enabled practitioners to calculate the severity of the alternatives to custody they should propose to the courts; the *combination order*, ushered in by the 1991 CJA, which gave the courts flexibility in specifying the content of such alternatives; the *justice model*, which offered an ideologically acceptable rehabilitative practice; the requirement upon practitioners, under the 1991 Act, to assess the *dangerousness and future risk* posed by the offender; and longer periods of toughened *post-release supervision*. The 'new penology' represented a merging of managerial, technical and social scientific discourses into a new technology for the optimal disposition of adjudicated offenders. As Feely and Simon observe:

> The new penology is neither about punishing nor rehabilitating individuals. It is about identifying and managing unruly groups. It is concerned with the rationality not of individual behaviour or even community organisation, but of managerial processes. It's goal is not to eliminate crime but to make it tolerable through systemic co-ordination. . . . For example, although parole and probation have long been justified as a means of reintegrating offenders into the community, increasingly they are being seen as cost-effective ways of imposing long-term management on the dangerous.
>
> (Feely and Simon 1992: 453–4)

This is where the fantasy world of the 'justice model' and the spurious new rehabilitations intersect with the reality of burgeoning crime and social deprivation in the poorest neighbourhoods. The new penology provides the means whereby the residents of these neighbourhoods are to be monitored, contained and, from time to time, disciplined. This task is made both more manageable and more urgent by their progressive social and economic isolation – what Davis (1990) describes as their 'South Africanisation'.

The youth justice lobby had chosen to remain silent about the growing poverty, victimisation and social polarisation occurring in the high-crime neighbourhoods from which the bulk of adjudicated young offenders were drawn. They had done so because of their fear that, if the issues of falling youth custody rates and burgeoning youth crime were brought together, a causal connection might be made, and a new 'crusade' against youth crime, emanating from the government's back benches and the media, might be set in train. By 1991 it appeared that their restraint was to be rewarded. The 1991 CJA marked the moment when the lessons learnt in the development of youth justice in the 1980s were to be enshrined in law and translated into the adult justice system. With this, the prize which had eluded penal reformers throughout the century, the cessation of the imprisonment of children under the age of 15, appeared to be almost within their grasp.

1992–1996: The crisis of political legitimacy and the repoliticisation of youth justice

However, this optimism was to be short-lived. In 1992 there were riots in Bristol, Salford and Burnley, which revived the anxieties generated by the 1991 riots in Oxford, Cardiff and Tyneside. In Manchester a 14-year-old bystander was shot dead in the Moss Side 'crack wars', and in London a 12-year-old was stabbed in his school playground. Ram-Raiding and Twocking were in the headlines, and John Major's Conservative government, recently weakened by a narrow electoral victory, was under attack from the Labour Party on its law-and-order record. Labour made great play of the fact that youth crime was running out of control and that the traditional 'party of law and order' was unwilling and unable to contain it. And then two-year-old James Bulger was brutally murdered by two truanting ten-year-olds. The political storm which accompanied this murder and the ensuing trial focused national attention on the government's capacity to discharge its most important responsibility and fulfil the primary rationale for its very existence, the maintenance of social order. The Major government was under growing pressure to find a new idea and a new policy.

The key reforms of the 1991 Criminal Justice Act were abandoned. In March 1993, only five months after the newly implemented Act had ended the imprisonment of children under 15, Kenneth Clarke, the Home Secretary, promised to create 200 places in new 'Secure Training Centres' for 12- to 15-year-olds. This *volte face* signalled a new era in which crime in general, and youth crime in particular, were to be repoliticised and moved back to the centre of the political stage. These changes dealt a severe blow to the depoliticised delinquency-management strategies of the 1980s.

Michael Howard replaced Kenneth Clarke as Home Secretary in July 1993, and within weeks he began putting his personal stamp upon youth justice policy. In October of that year, at the Conservative Party conference he propounded his belief that:

> Prison Works. It ensures that we are protected from murderers, muggers and rapists – and it makes many who are tempted to commit crime think twice. . . . This may mean that many more people will go to prison. I do not flinch from that. We shall no longer judge the success of our system of justice by a fall in our prison population.

Whereas Clarke was essentially a pragmatic hatchet man, ruthlessly cutting government expenditure as he was promoted from one government department to another, Howard was an ambitious, neo-conservative ideologue who took it upon himself to wage a populist war against the criminal justice and penal establishments. Howard's strategy involved placing himself consistently in breach of the law in order to precipitate high profile vote-winning confrontations with the courts and criminal justice agencies. In 1994 he set about toughening the Probation Service, by allowing direct recruitment of ex-NCOs and police officers and severing probation's traditional links with social-work education. Taking inspiration from some of the more punitive practices within the US correctional system, in February 1995 he announced plans for 'tougher and more demanding' 'house-of-pain' regimes, 'aimed at knocking criminal tendencies out of young offenders' (*The Times*, 5 February 1995). Between 1992 and 1995 the numbers of juveniles sentenced to custody rose from 3,900 to 5,100 (Home Office 1996).With this melange of toughened teenage prison regimes and new rehabilitations enshrined in a new, more restrictive and more punitive Criminal Justice Act, Howard hoped to restore the government's political legitimacy and the Conservative Party's electoral fortunes.

FRANCE: YOUTH CRIME AS A CRISIS OF CITIZENSHIP

In 1981 approximately 3,500,000 offences were recorded by the police in both Britain and France. Both countries had witnessed steady increases in recorded crime in general, and recorded youth crime in particular, and both confronted youth riots on the streets of their major cities. However, by the end of the 1980s the number of offences recorded in Britain was approaching 6,000,000 while in France, between 1983 and 1986 there was a decline in recorded offences to around 3,000,000, where it remained for the rest of the decade (Parti Socialiste Français 1986; De Liège 1991; Home Office 1994). In Britain crime appears to have risen fastest in the poorest neighbourhoods (Hope 1994). However, in France it was in the poorest neighbourhoods that the fall in the crime rate was most marked (King 1989; De Liège 1991).

As the 1980s progressed, youth justice policy in Britain developed a narrowly focused concern with the operation of the apparatus of justice. In France during the same period, policies inspired by governmental concerns about the erosion of social cohesion, culminated in the development of a complex national 'social prevention' programme. This brought together politicians, professionals and citizen groups at national, regional and local levels in a programme which linked concerns about poverty, drugs, mental health, educational attainment, racial conflict and unemployment with questions of crime and social disorder.

Cooling out the long hot summer

Upon its election in 1981 the socialist administration of François Mitterrand faced nation-wide riots in the multi-racial *banlieues*. Fearing that they might reach the proportions they had attained in Britain, Mitterrand established the *étés jeunes*, a 100,000-strong national summer play scheme, and established a commission of town mayors under the chairmanship of Henri Bonnemaison. The Bonnemaison Commission, which brought together both Gaullist and Socialist mayors to devise a national strategy produced its report, *Face à la délinquence: prévention, répression, solidarité*, in 1983. The report asserted that if effective action against the causes of crime was to be taken, a policy was needed that was flexible, adapted to local circumstances, and structurally connected with the activities of government departments and local authorities, the judiciary, the voluntary sector and the needs and wishes of citizens (Bonnemaison Report 1983).

On the face of it, Bonnemaison was concerned with the effects of 'social exclusion' and the development of techniques of 'social prevention'. However, the commission was the central prop of a broader political initiative which aimed to revitalise a sense of 'citizenship' through the democratisation of those parts of the Republic where this sense was perceived to be most tenuous. This, Wieviorka (1994) notes, was deemed politically necessary because French society was perceived by the Socialists to have undergone 'une grande mutation' in the previous two decades. This 'mutation' was characterised by the dissipation of industrial society and the working-class movement, the supplanting of collectivism by individualism and subjectivism, mass unemployment and racial conflict. It was also evident to the Mitterrand administration that the multi-racial *banlieue*, the site of the 1981 riots, was the place *par excellence* where this sense of citizenship was at its weakest. The Bonnemaison Commission was not, therefore, solely concerned with the prevention of crime, but with the prevention of those forms of social marginalisation or exclusion which threatened social cohesion and social order, and hence the political legitimacy of the Republic. Thus, in its report, the Commission argued that if youth crime and disorder in the *banlieues* were to be curbed, the solution must lie in a process of political incorporation, an expression of *solidarité* with the people who lived there (King 1989).

The structure of the social prevention programme

At a national level, the National Council for the Prevention of Delinquency, chaired by the Prime Minister and attended by the majority of town mayors and representatives from the relevant government ministries, was established in June 1983. At regional level, Councils for the Prevention of Crime chaired by the chief civil servant (the Commissaire de la République) with the Chief Judicial Officer (the Procureur de la République) as the vice-chair, were established. At local level, Communal Councils for the Prevention of Crime, chaired by the town mayors were established. Communal Councils monitored local youth crime patterns, established special working groups to deal with particular problems and targeted central government funds on these problems. Their 'arms and legs' were *animateurs sociales* who worked at face-to-face level with local young people, and latterly adults, to devise local solutions to local problems. Graham and Bennett (1995) note that:

> The main aim of the Communal Council is to reduce crime through improving the urban environment, reducing unemployment

among the young, improving facilities for education and training, combating racial discrimination and encouraging the assimilation and integration of marginalised groups, particularly alienated youngsters and immigrants. To facilitate this process, a national network of Youth Centres, known as *Missions Locales* has been set up in more than 100 towns and cities. These centres try to bridge the transition between school and work for the unemployed and the unqualified (aged 16–25) by offering youth training and advice and assistance on matters such as improving literacy, managing financial affairs and finding accommodation. They also encourage young people, particularly the unemployed, to set up and run their own projects.

(Graham and Bennett 1993: 135)

This structure maximised information exchange, enabled the horizontal co-ordination of neighbourhoods and local agencies and the vertical co-ordination of neighbourhoods with central government agencies and departments (De Liège 1991). Importantly, it also ensured that political 'feedback loops' were created between the poorest neighbourhoods and the office of the Prime Minister.

What set the Mitterrand Social Prevention Initiative apart from previous initiatives in France and elsewhere was the precision with which neighbourhoods and young people were targeted for intervention.

With the new government, specific practices were identified and roles apportioned within the local communities and their municipal or district representatives. Within these local contexts, an initial phase of consultation was expected to deliver a 'security diagnosis'. This preliminary joint exercise had the purpose of assessing the needs and problems of specific areas.

(Gallo 1995: 76)

The structure of the initiative was developed in tandem with a dual strategy of *decentralisation* – the creation of new regional and departmental bodies headed by elected officials – and *deconcentration* – in which departmental and regional prefects, and other local officials of central government, were granted much greater autonomy – and a *politique de la ville* which was gradually developed through the 1980s (Le Gales 1994; Lemierre 1994). (In Britain during the same period local democracy was being progressively weakened by the transfer of power, responsibilities and resources from local authorities to central government. (Hutton 1995; Jenkins 1995)). Although the election in France of a government of the political Right in 1986 signalled reductions in the scale of the Social Prevention initiative, the new government affirmed its commitment to the programme. Thus, following the 1990 riots in Lyons and Paris, responsibility for crime prevention was handed to a newly created Minister of State for Cities.

This led to a sharpening of the focus upon urban crime and an attempt to involve the private sector in crime prevention to a far greater degree. The Praedrie Report *Enterprises and Neighbourhoods* (1991) observed that, if the *banlieues* were to be successfully drawn into the economic mainstream, they would require much greater involvement with, and much more investment from, the business community and far better communication between those in need of employment and those in need of workers. As a result, in 1992, a National Foundation for Integration was established by a consortium of industrialists, supported by the government, which offered financial incentives to firms investing in neighbourhoods with high levels of social and economic need. Because, in France, policy was developed at national level in consultation with the Ministries of Justice, Housing, Health and Social Affairs, the structure of inter-professional and inter-agency co-operation at a local level, the roles played by public professionals and the resources to be devoted to the discharge of these roles were determined nationally, as was the space for negotiation between elected officials, administrators and citizen groups.

Youth justice

In France youth justice and child care and protection are both the responsibility of DPJJ (*Direction de la Protection Judiciare et de la Jeunesse*). DPJJ trains and employs all the children's judges and court social workers in France. It works through its *Action Educative* bureaux (akin to off-site units) with children who are unwilling or unable to stay in mainstream schooling. It employs over 1,000 detached/outreach youth workers and has been a lead agency in the development of the Social Prevention initiative at a local level.

Unlike the UK, youth justice in France is deeply imbued with 'welfarist' assumptions about the origins of, and solutions to, the problem of youth crime. However, whereas in the UK 'welfarism' tends to be associated with a preoccupation with family functioning, DPJJ social workers are required to work collaboratively with other individuals, groups, organisations and agencies to enhance the educational and vocational opportunities available to socially disadvantaged children and their families and the quality of life within their neighbourhoods (Ely and Stanley 1990; Cooper *et al.* 1995).

As we have seen, in England and Wales in the 1980s youth justice workers effectively abandoned the attempt to address the social factors deemed to be associated with youth crime, in favour of more narrowly focused delinquency-management strategies aimed at diverting children and young people from the justice system. In France, by contrast, DPJJ social workers have been at the forefront of the attempt to elaborate new forms of social intervention. This has been easier for DPJJ workers than for some other social workers in other agencies however. Over the period, the involvement of social work in the Social Prevention initiative has led to a redefinition of the social-work role and a refocusing of the social-work task. This has led, in some cases, to the recruitment of new personnel with new skills and perspectives and the construction of new political alliances (Picard 1995). Crescy Cannan (1996) has observed that some social workers found involvement in collective action with neighbourhood groups difficult, preferring to play a more traditional role with individual service users. As a result, some *départements* and *communes* have grown impatient with professional social work's reluctance to grasp the new roles and have employed people like sociologists and geographers, who have been more attuned to the goals of the Social Prevention initiative.

A TALE OF TWO HOUSING ESTATES

Between 1993 and 1995 I was involved in a study of the responses of public professionals, politicians and local residents to youth crime and the violent victimisation of children and young people on the Dickens Estate in east London and the Flaubert Estate in an industrial suburb to the west of Paris (Pearce 1995; Pitts 1995). In many ways the two estates typified the changing pattern of crime and victimisation, and changing professional responses to it, in the two countries in this period. Whereas on the Flaubert Estate there has been a sustained attempt, since 1983, to develop a coherent political and professional response to these problems, on the Dickens Estate the picture was different. During our research violence, particularly racial violence, on the estate had reached record levels, making it the most violent neighbourhood in a traditionally high-crime London borough. The Flaubert Estate, having topped the French youth crime league in the early 1980s, now had a level of crime and violence somewhat below the national average. The following vignettes suggest some of the key differences in the responses of public professionals, politicians and local residents to youth crime and disorder on the two estates. It is the argument of this chapter that these differences were a product of two quite different policy responses to the problem of youth crime and social and economic exclusion by national governments.

Housing

Flaubert

Housing policy aimed to locate the children and relatives of local residents in local accommodation in order to strengthen ties of friendship and kinship, stabilise the neighbourhood and strengthen indigenous sources of social control. This was decided by the locally elected Neighbourhood Council, which was established, through negotiations with the mayor's office, as an additional tier of local government in the *quartier* in the late 1980s. All residents of 16 and over, irrespective of immigration status, were allowed to vote for the Neighbourhood Council, and around 40 per cent did. Seventy-five per cent of the population of the Flaubert Estate were of north African, central African, Turkish or Portuguese origin, and most had never voted before in any French election. As a result of this policy, however, many apartments were overcrowded, being unsuitable for the many large families on the estate. However new, larger, council homes and a new hospital are now being constructed alongside the estate. The Neighbourhood Council had previously initiated a project with the mayor's office in which consecrated rooms were established at the town abattoir where Islamic religious rites could be practised. One of the consequences of these developments had been that requests for transfers off the estate had dwindled, while the waiting list for transfers onto the estate had grown significantly.

Dickens

The Housing Department operated a system of housing priority points, determined on the basis of social need. This was a policy which was increasingly difficult to implement in the face of the erosion of good-quality local housing stock occasioned by central government's 'right to buy' strategy. This meant that 'disruptive' tenants – those who did not pay their rent regularly, the homeless (often young single-parent and Bengali families) and successive waves of refugees – were allocated to the unpopular and underused tower blocks on the estate which were notorious for their high crime rate and drug-dealing. This had produced a less stable neighbourhood with fewer ties of kinship and friendship. One of the consequences of this was that the neighbourhood had one of the highest levels of racial attacks in the borough, and support for the National Front amongst established white families was strong.

Employment

Flaubert

Local employment policy aimed to offer local jobs in the public and voluntary sectors to local people in order to reduce local unemployment and promote interaction between neighbours. The policy was developed by the Local Authority in liaison with the Neighbourhood Council, the social workers of DPJJ, the *Mission Locale* and a national voluntary youth welfare and training agency *Association Jeunesse, Culture, Loisirs, Technique* (JCLT). JCLT developed long-term youth and adult training, an extensive programme of social and cultural activities and operated a residential *foyer* for children and young people from the neighbourhood who were unable to live with their families. JCLT was also commissioned by the Ministry of Social Affairs to administer, locally, the *Revenue Minimum d'Insertion*, introduced in 1988 to provide income maintenance and counselling and advice for unemployed young people. Professional workers recognised that racism and the poor reputation of the estate often made it difficult to place people in employment beyond the estate, but their emphasis on extended periods of training leading to nationally recognised qualifications meant that they had achieved some success in equipping trainees for higher paid, skilled, work in the *département* and in Paris.

Dickens

Previous employment initiatives on the estate had reduced levels of violence while in operation. However, during the research there were no specific training or employment initiatives in operation on the estate, a problem exacerbated by the transfer of responsibility for youth training to employers and the cessation of income support.

Education

Flaubert

On the basis of national educational 'league tables', the estate had been designated a *zone éducationale prioritaire* by the French Ministry of Education. This meant that additional resources had been directed towards the schools in the neighbourhood. These included additional specialist staff, additional staff hours for after-school work and the construction of a radio station which provided public-service broadcasting to the surrounding region, in an attempt to form closer and more positive social and economic links. In tandem with these initiatives, *Femmes Relais*, a semi-formal community organisation, comprising Senegalese, north African, Kurdish, Iranian and Portuguese mothers, supported by Maghrebian community workers from the Mayor's Office, met regularly with representatives of the school, the police, and the local administration to discuss the problems confronting young people; drugs, violence, racism, under-achievement, truancy, bullying, etc., in the school and in the neighbourhood, and to devise collaborative, corporate, solutions. *Femmes Relais*, in conjunction with JCLT, also offered language tuition and vocational training to parents. Meanwhile, local young people undertaking national service had been recruited by the school as 'mentors' and 'recreational counsellors'. They also provided surveillance and protection against victimisation for school students and had had the effect of reducing student–student violence significantly.

Dickens

Levels of attainment in the secondary school on the Dickens Estate were roughly similar to those in the secondary school on the Flaubert Estate, *vis-à-vis* the national average. However, the implementation of the National Curriculum and Local Management of Schools had generated an enormously increased administrative load which made it increasingly difficult for the school to provide the requisite pastoral, sporting and social activities. These pressures were placing at risk the very close staff–student relationships and high standards of pastoral care for which the school was renowned. Increasingly the school was becoming the locus and focus for violent racial conflict which spilt over from the neighbourhood. A few low-achieving white boys, those most likely to be the perpetrators of racial violence, continued to pose a serious problem to the school, and (largely as a result of the pressures identified above) staff were resorting to exclusion more frequently. These students felt marginalised and scapegoated, and exclusion appeared to deepen their frustration and anger. School students who were victimised – particularly Bengali children and young people – tended not to tell their parents, partly because they were concerned not to add to their parents' worries and partly because the only recourse available to parents was to stop their children going out. As a result, youngsters often opted to say nothing to the adults around them whom they perceived as being more or less powerless in the situation. The school, like others in adjacent areas, had attempted to respond to these difficulties by developing a Parent-Teacher Association, but mistrust amongst some Bengali parents, and an apparent lack of interest amongst many others, had confounded its efforts. However, despite the formidable problems with which the school was attempting to wrestle, rather than the promise of additional support and resources, staff were 'motivated' by the threat of a Ministry of Education hit squad intervening if standards fell further.

Inter-agency co-operation

Flaubert

Official initiatives to reduce victimisation through inter-agency and interprofessional collaboration had been established since the early 1980s. The mayor had been central to this process, and the arrangements for co-operation grew out of protracted and continuing negotiations between him and his fellow politicians and representatives of the adults and young people on the estate (Le Gales 1994; Jazouli 1995; Picard 1995). As we have noted, these negotiations had spawned the Neighbourhood Council. For its part, central government required statutory and voluntary welfare agencies, as a condition of their funding, to collaborate in projects which aimed to resolve problems of community life and neighbourhood conflict. They were required, in particular, to focus upon problems of social marginality, 'exclusion', and to promote 'inclusion' via activities which contributed to the 'insertion' of young people into significant educational and vocational opportunities. These inter-agency and interprofessional initiatives had been institutionalised into the day-to-day practices of statutory and voluntary agencies in the neighbourhood. At the time of our research, this complex collaborative network had been evolving for eleven years.

Dickens

Public professionals from statutory agencies felt themselves to be under pressure to reconcile their commitment to inter-agency and interprofessional co-operation with their statutory responsibilities. In the context of steadily reducing Local Authority budgets, inter-agency co-operation sometimes became another means whereby agencies would attempt to discharge or displace their statutory responsibilities. Agency priorities tended to be determined by their own 'mission statements' or 'quality targets', and even when problems of neighbourhood conflict were articulated, they seldom found their way onto agency 'agendas'. In the fields of child protection and youth justice, workers experienced an annexation of the professional task, as they pursued priorities and discharged functions specified in ever greater detail by central government departments. This caused senior officers of the relevant departments to observe that the only response available to the council in the case of an incident of racial violence directed against a child or young person was to make the victim the subject of a child-protection investigation, and to subject the perpetrator, if apprehended, to a correctional programme at the council's Youth Justice Centre. The professionals involved knew that this individualisation of a profoundly social and political conflict was wholly inadequate, but they felt that they no longer had the means to engage with social conflict in the public domain.

Beyond this, some public professionals on the Dickens Estate were reluctant to involve the 'public' in those problem-solving processes which did exist, because to do so would necessarily bring them into confrontation with deep-rooted inter-communal conflicts. Thus, problem-solving tended to be left to the professionals. Crime-prevention programmes, 'Safer Neighbourhoods', 'Safer Cities', etc., had come and gone, having some effect while they lasted but – because they were never seriously planned to mesh with the practices of local agencies – they had little lasting impact. As a result, both professionals and local people had grown cynical about such short-term initiatives. Increasingly, agencies found themselves in competition for dwindling central government crime-prevention resources, which limited still further their motivation and capacity to collaborate.

Crime prevention, youth justice and the courts

Flaubert

Political, administrative and judicial systems tended to work together to render youth justice responsive to local situational, social, economic and cultural factors which might precipitate youth crime and victimisation. Social prevention initiatives were institutionalised and integrated within and between Local Authority departments, locally-based offices of central government, central government departments, the voluntary sector and the 'youth justice system'. French children's judges are state employees, and they are expected to be active in their neighbourhoods, using knowledge gained through dealing with child care and juvenile offending cases to help focus the efforts and develop the activities of local welfare, educational, training and employment agencies. They are also enjoined to promote social 'insertion' as a way of reducing crime and public disorder. On the Flaubert Estate they were pursuing these objectives through their membership of the management committees of local voluntary and neighbourhood organisations and through regular meetings with the staff of DPJJ.

Dickens

On the Dickens Estate there was a clear separation between local crime-prevention initiatives, which incorporated some 'social', but mainly 'situational', elements, and the Local Authority youth justice service, which was wedded to an offence-focused 'delinquency-management' strategy. Crime-prevention initiatives on the estate had been time-limited and project-based. They were therefore extra, rather than integral, to the services provided locally by statutory and voluntary agencies. The magistrates approached during the research chose not to participate. Although they had sentenced young people and adults from the neighbourhood, not infrequently for racially motivated crimes and gang-fighting, they claimed to be insufficiently familiar with the neighbourhood and its problems to be of any help to the research team.

Local politics

Flaubert

The mayor of the suburb in which the Flaubert Estate is built, like the majority of town mayors in France, served on the *Conseil National de Prevention de la Délinquence* chaired by the French Prime Minister. The Mayor's Office co-ordinates the expenditure of the town's share of the national Urban Policy budget with national, local and EU funds. The town has constructed a young people's resource centre, the Pagoda, on the Flaubert Estate, where the mayor and his representatives met local people once a month to discuss problems of community life in general and the predicament of young people on the estate in particular. As such, the Mayor's Office served as a political link between the 'private troubles' of the residents of the Estate and the 'public issues' which formed the basis for the development of urban policy at a national level.

Dickens

The dominant Labour group on the council was at odds with both Government policy and the ideas espoused by the national party's front bench. At the time of our research it was recentralising the services which had been 'localised' by the previous Liberal Democrat administration. Very little information about this process had reached the electorate at this point. A sustained attempt by the secondary school on the Dickens Estate to involve local councillors in discussions about the safety of school students had proved ineffective.

A POLITICISED PRACTICE

In contrasting these two neighbourhoods we encounter one in which a politically engaged public is devising new forms of social solidarity and another in which social atomisation is accelerating. These differences have little to do with the proclivities or potential of local residents, or the skills and abilities of the public professionals who serve them. Rather they speak to the social and political possibilities which can be opened-up by a belief among politicians that social cohesion matters.

Not since the American Poverty Programme of the 1960s has there been a governmental assault upon the problem of social cohesion on the scale of the French Social Prevention initiative of the 1980s. The American Poverty Programme, orchestrated by the Kennedy and Johnson administrations, aimed to circumvent existing political and administrative structures and provide alternative vehicles for political participation amongst the poor (Marris and Rein 1967; Moynihan 1969; Cloward and Fox-Piven 1972). Like the neo-conservatives of the 1980s and 1990s, the architects of the American Poverty Programme located the problem in hidebound, oppressive and self-serving state services and bureaucracies which, while claiming to ameliorate the condition of the poor, merely compounded it. In pursuing the consequences of this analysis, however, the state found itself in a situation which was both unprecedented and extremely uncomfortable, since it effectively sanctioned the expenditure of central government funds on the subversion of local government.

The ensuing popular protests and riots notwithstanding, the alternative structures developed in the struggle against the 'establishment' were never integral to the processes of political decision-making and social change. Although these alternative structures offered some members of the indigenous Black leadership a means of entering an emergent Black middle class, they failed to institutionalise mechanisms whereby the bulk of the poor, who were Black and Hispanic, could be reconnected with the organised working class, which was predominantly White (Wilson 1987). In the end therefore, as Cloward and Fox-Piven (1972) have argued, 'relief-giving turned out to be the most expeditious way to deal with the political pressure created by a dislocated poor, just as it had been many times in the past' (p. 256).

The French initiative of the 1980s emerged from a different political tradition, adopted a radically different political strategy and, in consequence, had a different effect upon the relationship between those on the social margins and the state. At the core of the political culture of both the USA and the UK is a notion of the state as a potentially antagonistic force, which, unless it is rigorously controlled, may at any moment encroach upon the lives and arrogate the liberties of citizens. Thus 'freedom' consists in minimising the role of the state. In France, and many other western European states, by contrast, the state is conceived as a potentially creative force, constituted by, and representative of, the collective interest of its citizens. Although both these views are idealisations, they open doors to quite different political possibilities for governments trying to fashion responses to the problems of crime and social cohesion.

Rather than circumventing the state apparatus, the task defined by Mitterrand and Bonnemaison concerned the construction, and then the institutionalisation, of a new relationship between the political centre and the social margins. This was to be achieved through the reform and co-ordination of the relevant ministries and a devolution of state power which aimed to repoliticise. democratise, and localise key areas of state activity and transform the practices of their agents. In consequence, for a time, the French initiative achieved the prize which had eluded the Kennedy and Johnson administrations: the construction of a political 'hot line' between the Head of State and the ghetto.

Although the French initiative adopted many of the techniques pioneered in the American poverty programme, it was designed to solve the very different social and economic problems of the 1980s. The American poverty programme of the 1960s and 1970s aimed to break down the political, educational, bureaucratic and racial barriers which excluded the poor from full participation in a traditional, three-tier, class structure in an expanding economy. The French initiative of the 1980s was borne of a recognition that economic globalisation and a burgeoning new technology had transformed class relations, and that now the key social division was between a contracting, relatively prosperous and skilled workforce and the growing body of people (usually young and often non-White) who appeared to be permanently excluded from economic activity altogether (Donzelot and Roman 1991; Wilson 1987).

The social and political analysis upon which the French initiative was based marked an early recognition of the forces which were transforming advanced industrial societies throughout Europe and beyond. Its unique contribution was to devise new forms of social solidarity, and new routes to citizenship, to replace traditional but defunct social and political structures rooted in the work-place. Its other unique features were the precision of its aims and the exhaustiveness and inclusiveness of the process by which those aims were arrived at. Its objectives were clearly specified, and the interventions to which they gave rise were targeted precisely on the basis of detailed local assessments (Gallo 1995).

The painstaking construction of the French Social Prevention initiative bore fruit at neighbourhood level. On the Dickens Estate, the social and economic forces making for destabilisation had proceeded unchecked by central or local government. On the Flaubert Estate, the economic interventions – the opening-up of primary-sector employment opportunities beyond the estate by the *Mission Locale*, the local housing strategies devised by the Neighbourhood Council, the training initiatives of JCLT, the social action and anti-racist programmes of the DPJJ – were co-ordinated by the Mayor's Office. This meant that a housing strategy that located several generations of the same family in close proximity articulated with an employment strategy that, by placing local young people and adults together in work groups on the estate, reinforced relationships between the generations and created a higher degree of social interaction and mutual dependence between residents. These initiatives grew out of, and articulated with, negotiations between the mayor the Neighbourhood Council, *Femmes Relais*, and the 'socially excluded' young people of the estate whom the mayor met at his monthly meetings at the Pagoda.

The notion of 'social exclusion' has not really taken root in Anglo-Saxon academic and political debate, where the concept of the 'underclass' has achieved greater currency. The term was introduced into the debate by William Julius Wilson (1987) in an attempt to demarcate, conceptually, those who had dropped through the bottom of the three-tier class structure. For Wilson this underclass comprises the long-term unemployed, the persistent poor, the denizens of the 'ghetto' who have lost regular and guaranteed access to markets (especially the labour market) and effective political representation. In Anglo-Saxon discourse the destiny of the underclass is inextricably linked to its role in the labour market. For commentators like Ralph Dahrendorf (1994), for example, exclusion from the labour market is assumed to place people virtually outside society. Yet, on the Flaubert Estate, through political and social action, disparate groups of people, previously effectively expelled from the economic and cultural mainstream, were successfully forged into a complex political constituency. Their common and separate interests were articulated through the new social and political structures, operating beyond the workplace, within and between local and central government, which were brought into being by the Social Prevention initiative.

The class structures in Britain and France have changed dramatically in the past twenty five years as tendencies towards social and economic polarisation have grown. However, in Britain in the 1980s and 1990s we witnessed a sustained attempt to separate questions of social class from questions of social inequality. In neo-conservative dogma, growing social inequality emerges as an inevitable, and desirable, consequence of economic deregulation, which is said to have opened up new economic opportunities for all, irrespective of social class. Thus, economic inequality is presented as a force promoting social equality, because it frees us from the redundant class divisions and class antagonisms which had previously imprisoned the entrepreneurial spirit of the nation. In practice, of course, the period was characterised by an even greater concentration of wealth and power, and deepening social divisions.

The French Social Prevention Initiative, by contrast, strove to counter tendencies towards social and economic polarisation by developing new bases for social solidarity in a post-Fordist society, through the devolution of political power and active intervention in the economy and the market. But did this represent a movement towards classlessness? That the French initiative was instrumental in redistributing some political power and some educational and vocational opportunity in favour of the poor is beyond dispute. That it therefore achieved some success in integrating previously excluded social groups into the social and economic mainstream is also evident. That that economic mainstream is characterised by deep class, gender and racial divisions is undeniable. Thus we can say that the French initiative has been conservative, insofar as it has helped to preserve and stabilise pre-existing social relations, and progressive, insofar as it has established new forms of political inclusion and new modes of political expression for populations which were previously effectively excluded from the political process.

Should a future British government wish to achieve a more just and harmonious society – or, indeed, if it simply wished to reduce crime – what, practically, might it do? It would probably strive to offer a stake in society to those who have none through the repoliticisation of local government and the development of educational and vocational opportunity in the poorest neighbourhoods. It would therefore have a direct interest in the simultaneous revitalisation of 'communities' and local economies in order to put an end to the chronic waste of human lives which structural youth unemployment represents, and to reduce the burgeoning costs of the crime and disorder it generates. If a future British government really wanted to do this, then the French Social Prevention initiative provides some intriguing answers but also, and perhaps more importantly, some crucially important questions about the basis of citizenship, participative democracy and social relations in a post-Fordist society. To date, however, these are questions which few British politicians have had the nerve to ask.

REFERENCES

Bonnemaison Report (1983) *Face a la délinquence: prévention, répression, solidarité: Rapport au premier ministre de la Commission des maires sur la securité*, Paris: La Documentation Française.

Cannan, C. (1996) 'The Impact of Social Development and Anti-Exclusion Policies on the French Social Work Professions', *Social Work in Europe* 3(2): 1–4.

Clarke, J., Cochrane, A. and McLaughlin E. (1994) *Managing Social Policy*, London: Sage Publications.

Cloward, R. and Fox-Piven, F. (1972) *Regulating the Poor: The Functions of Public Welfare,* London: Tavistock Publications.

Cooper, A., Hetherington, R., Baistow, K., Pitts, J. and Spriggs, A. (1995) *Positive Child Protection: A View From Abroad* Lyme Regis: Russell House Publishing.

Currie, E. (1991) 'International developments in crime and social policy', in NACRO, *Crime and Public Policy*, London: NACRO.

Dahrendorf, R. (1994) 'The changing quality of citizenship', in B. Van Steenbergen (ed.) *The Condition of Citizenship*, London: Sage Publications.

Davis, M. (1990) *City of Quartz*, London: Verso.

De Liège, M-P. (1991) 'Social development and the prevention of crime in France: A challenge for local parties and central government', in M. Farrell and F. Heidensohn *Crime in Europe* London: Routledge.

Donzelot, J. and Roman, J. (1991) 'Le déplacement de la question social', in J. Donzelot (ed.) *Face à l'exclusion*, Paris: Editions Espirit.

Ely, P. and Stanley, C. (1990) *The French Alternative: Delinquency Prevention and Child Protection in France*, London: NACRO.

Feeley, M. and Simon, J. (1992) 'The new penology: Notes on the emerging strategy of corrections and its implementation', *Criminology* 30(4): 452–74.

Forrester, D., Chatterton, M. and Pease, K. (1988) *The Kirkholt Burglary Prevention Project, Rochdale*, Crime Prevention Unit Paper 13, London: Home Office.

Gallo, E. (1995) 'The penal system in France: From correctionalism to managerialism', in V. Ruggerio, M. Ryan and J. Sim (eds) *Western*

European Penal Systems: A Critical Anatomy, London: Sage Publications.

Graham, J. and Bennett, T. (1993) *Crime Prevention Strategies in Europe and North America*, Helsinki: European Institute for Crime Prevention.

Graham, J. and Bowling, B. (1995) *Young People and Crime*, London: HMSO.

Graham, J. (1993) 'Crime prevention policies in Europe', *European Journal of Crime, Criminal Law and Criminal Justice* 1(2).

Hagan, J. (1993) 'The social embededness of crime and unemployment', *Criminology* 31: 455–91.

Hagell, A. and Newburn, T, (1994) *Persistent Young Offenders*, London: Policy Studies Institute.

Hall, S. (ed.) (1978) *Thatcherism*, London: New Left Review.

Home Office (1994) *The Criminal Statistics*, London: HMSO.

—— (1996) *Home Office Statistical Bulletin*, London: Home Office.

Hope, T. (1994) *Communities, Crime and Inequality in England and Wales*, paper presented to the 1994 Cropwood Round Table Conference *Preventing Crime and Disorder* Cambridge, Sept. 14–15.

—— (1995) 'Inequality and the future of community crime prevention', in S. P. Lab *Crime Prevention at a Crossroads*, American Academy of Criminal Justice Sciences Monograph Series, Cincinnati, OH: Anderson Publishing.

Hope, T. and Foster, J. (1992) 'Conflicting forces: Changing the dynamics of crime and community on a problem estate', *British Journal of Criminology* 32(92): 488–504.

Hutton ,W. (1995) *The State We're In*, London: Jonathan Cape.

Jazouli, A. (1995) *Une saison en banlieue,* Paris: Plon.

Jenkins, S. (1995) *Accountable to None: The Tory Nationalisation of Britain*, London: Hamish Hamilton.

King, M. (1989) 'Social Crime Prevention à la Thatcher', *Howard Journal* 28: 291–312

Lea, J. and Young, J. (1984) *What is to be Done About Law and Order*, Harmondsworth: Penguin.

Le Gales, P. (1994) 'The political dynamics of European policy implementation: Poverty III in Mantes-la-Jolie', *Local Government Policy Making* 20(5), May: 39–44.

Le Grand, J. (1996) 'Quasi-markets in welfare' in S. Trevillion and P. Beresford *Social Work Education and the Community Care Revolution*, London: NISW.

Lemierre, R. (1994) 'Juvenile services of the French Ministry of Justice', *Social Work in Europe* 1(2).

McGahey, R. (1986) 'Economic conditions, neighbourhood organisation and urban crime', in J.A. Reiss and M. Tonry *Communities and Crime*, Chicago: Chicago University Press.

Marris, P. and Rein, M. (1967) *Dilemmas of Social Reform: Poverty and Community Action in the United States,* New York: Atherton Press.

Mills, C.W. (1957) *The Sociological Imagination*, Harmondsworth: Penguin.

Moynihan, D. P. (1969) *Maximum Feasible Misunderstanding: Community Action in the War on Poverty*, New York: Free Press.

Page, D. (1993) *Building for Communities: a Study of New Housing Association Estates*, York: Joseph Rowntree Foundation.

Parti Socialiste Français (1986) *Les murs d'argent: Manifeste contre la privatisation des prisons*, Paris: Parti Socialiste.

Pearce, J. J. (1995) 'French lessons: Young people comparative research and community safety', *Social Work in Europe* 1(3): 32–6.

Picard, P. (1995) *Mantes-la-jolie: Carnet de route d'un mairie de banlieue*, Paris: Syros

Pitts, J. (1995) 'Public issues and private troubles: A tale of two cities', *Social Work in Europe* 2(1): 3–11.

—— (1996) 'The politics and practice of youth justice', in E. McLaughlin. and J. Muncie (eds), *Controlling Crime*, London: Sage Publications/Open University Press.

Rowntree Foundation (1996) *The Future of Work: Contributions to the Debate*, York: Joseph Rowntree Foundation.

Scull, A. (1977) *Decarceration*, New Jersey: Spectrum Books.

Thorpe, D., Smith, D., Green, C. and Paley, J. (1980) *Out of Care* London: Allen and Unwin.

Wieviorka, M. (1994) 'Racism in Europe: Unity and diversity', in A. Ratsani and S. Westwood *Racism, Modernity, Identity on the Western Front*, Cambridge: Polity Press.

Wilson, W. J. (1987) *The Truly Disadvantaged: the Inner City, the Underclass and Public Policy*, Chicago: University of Chicago Press.

Chapter 8

Young single mothers

Robert Page

INTRODUCTION

The issue of lone motherhood has returned towards the top of the political and social agenda in recent years, not least because of concerted media attention. For example, in the autumn of 1996 one national newspaper published a large front-page picture of a 13-year-old mother cradling her 15-day-old baby, describing it as a 'poignant image that sums up the moral confusion facing Britain today' (*Express*, 29 October 1996). In an era in which attention is being focused on social fragmentation, rising crime rates and the growth in 'welfare' dependence, it is not surprising to find the spotlight falling on lone mothers. Lone motherhood is being viewed as increasingly problematic for society – on the grounds that it occurs more as a result of deliberate or inappropriate personal choice than as a result of misfortune, and that it is an economically precarious family formation and inimical to the appropriate socialisation of children. In a sense, the young single mother has become a potent symbol of what many regard as a deep-rooted malaise in British society. In such a climate it is difficult to see how young single mothers will be accorded full membership of a classless society. Indeed, current policy initiatives appear to be based on the assumption that single mothers should be stigmatised and excluded, rather than integrated into society. Before examining contemporary debates about young single motherhood, it is useful to look briefly at the treatment of this group over time, in order to give some context to the theme of 'classlessness'.

THE HISTORICAL BACKCLOTH

The single or unmarried mother has been the subject of public concern over the centuries because hers is a form of parenthood associated with immorality, public dependence and social instability.

The moral transgressor

By engaging in sexual relations before marriage and giving birth to an 'illegitimate' child, single mothers were seen to pose a threat to Christian ideals of marriage and family life. Unmarried mothers were liable to be brought before the Ecclesiastical courts to answer charges of incontinence (a term which covered both fornication and adultery) and bastardy. Those convicted were usually required to undergo some form of penance – the severity of which varied according to the nature of the offence (Helmholz 1975). For example, one mother convicted of bastardy in Kent in the mid-sixteenth century was ordered to stand before her local church congregation 'in her petticoat with a white sheet about her' while the priest delivered 'the whole homily of adultery' (Emmison 1973: 12).

While it is difficult to gauge the impact of such sanctions on transgressors or prospective miscreants (Hair 1966; 1970), there is some evidence to suggest that fear of disgrace led some unmarried women to abort their child or 'dispose' of it shortly after birth (Macfarlane 1980). The fact that there was a separate ecclesiastical offence of harbouring an unwed mother also lends support to the view that attempts were made to avoid the shame of 'disclosure'. For example, in 1564 an East Horndon man who had sheltered a pregnant woman was sentenced to public penance in the market place and fined 2 shillings, while a curate who 'let his own daughter "go away unpunished" . . . was enjoined to confess that "he had offended God and the congregation in harbouring his daughter" ' (Emmison 1973: 27).

The Ecclesiastical courts declined in importance from around the latter part of sixteenth century (May 1930). Indeed, with the demise of shame punishments and the abolition of the offence of incontinence in the eighteenth century, the influence of the Ecclesiastical courts (though not of religion itself) had all but faded away. The shift from Ecclesiastical to a more secular jurisdiction did not, however, mean that the issue of single motherhood disappeared from the public sphere. Although there was less formal concern with morality *per se*, there was considerable interest in the financial costs associated with single motherhood.

The public dependent

In the period from 1500 to 1900 secular authorities at both local and national levels attempted to minimise the financial dependence of single mothers and their children. For example, public concern about the economic consequences of illegitimacy intensified in the post-feudal era, with the result that liable relatives were subjected to various forms of physical and monetary sanction. At the local level, officials used every means possible to discourage single-mother dependence, including the forcible removal of pregnant women to a neighbouring parish in order to prevent the child gaining 'legal' settlement.

The rapid rise in illegitimacy in the eighteenth century (Shorter 1977) – the precise reasons for which are difficult to disentangle (Laslett, *et al.* 1980) – led to further attempts to limit parish liability in this sphere. Poorer mothers were detained in Houses of Correction and, subsequently, in workhouses, which were frequently used as maternity wards for poor, homeless, pregnant women (Oxley 1974).

Although the growth of charitable activity in the eighteenth and nineteenth centuries brought about some improvement in the care afforded to single mothers (Owen 1965; Finlayson 1994), there was little change in public provision for this group. Following the 1834 Poor Law Amendment Act destitute single mothers were required to enter the workhouse, where they were often treated more harshly than other inmates (Anstruther 1973; Longmate 1974). Even those single mothers who were able to subsist outside the workhouse were often forced to leave their children with baby-farmers of questionable proficiency (Heywood 1978; Pinchbeck and Hewitt 1973).

In the early part of the twentieth century public policy for single mothers began to evolve in a more 'progressive' direction, not least because of the work of the National Council for the Unmarried Mother and her Child, which had been established in 1918. This organisation played a major role in highlighting the plight of single mothers, continually stressing the need for increased financial assistance if these mothers were to be afforded opportunities to bring up their children (Macaskill 1993).

The deficient parent

Concern has also been expressed about the parenting capabilities of young single mothers. As Smart (1996) notes, parenting 'standards' have changed over time. In earlier periods the avoidance of deliberate harm (infanticide or physical assault) was the principal focus of collective interest, whereas concern about the social and emotional nurturing of children has been a more recent development.

While the single mother has always had some form of 'legal' responsibility for her child (though the child itself had no legal standing) the issue of whether she should be encouraged, or even permitted, to raise her child has been resolved in varying ways over time. For example, single mothers who requested public assistance following the introduction of the Poor Law Amendment Act in 1834 were not permitted to receive outdoor relief but were required to enter the workhouse – an institutional arrangement which allowed economies of care to operate (one or two mothers could care for all the children, while the others could be set to work). Institutional care was also favoured by some early philanthropic bodies, which believed it offered the best prospects for rehabilitation, and by eugenicists concerned about the growth of 'feeble-minded' single motherhood (National Council for Civil Liberties 1951; Middleton 1971; Marks 1992).

The parenting skills of those mothers who were able to remain economically independent were, like working-class mothers in general, subject to ever-closer scrutiny as a result of the growing influence of philanthropic and state activity concerned with the physical well-being of children. Impoverished single mothers were likely to fall foul of these newly imposed standards of care which 'were extended to include the immense realm of the psychological care and nurture of the child' (Smart 1996: 46) after the Second World War (Bowlby 1965; Winnicott 1957). Although post-1945 single mothers were not intended to gain financially from the long-running campaign for the endowment of motherhood (Rathbone 1924; Macnicol 1980), they did benefit from a number of wartime welfare initiatives (Ferguson and Fitzgerald 1954; Middleton 1971), although their suitability as parents remained a matter of concern.

In an era in which unwanted conceptions could more easily be avoided (P. Clarke 1996: 217–21) it became fashionable to suggest that the pregnancy of single women was indicative of some form of psychological disturbance (Young 1954; Greenberg *et al.* 1959;

Eysenck 1961). Indeed, a number of researchers suggested that psychological dysfunction was even more likely to be found among those who decided to keep their children, rather than opting for either abortion or adoption (Naiman 1966, 1971; Floyd and Viney 1974; Yelloly 1965).

A number of post-1945 studies also highlighted the fact that young single mothers tended to come from culturally deficient working-class communities.

> Illegitimacy, like delinquency, thrives when social values, cultural, as well as material are low. Insecure family life, poor and overcrowded homes, lack of constructive recreational aims and outlets, lack of general planning ability, and permissive attitudes to extra-marital relations may all contribute to its occurrence.
>
> (Thompson 1956: 110)

These negative assessments of young single mothers undoubtedly had an impact on social work practice in the late 1940s and 1950s – an era in which adoption was often presented as the best, or even the only, option for young single mothers (Cheetham 1977; Vincent 1978; Page 1984; Spensky 1992).

SINGLE MOTHERHOOD IN THE POST-1945 ERA

Towards citizenship? Young single mothers during the 'welfare consensus' – from exclusion to partial inclusion?

In considering the position of the young single mother in the post-1945 era it is useful, first, to examine how this group fared during the so-called period of 'welfare consensus', from 1945 to the mid-1970s (Lowe 1990; Dutton 1991). Although it has been argued that the notion of a consensus is hard to sustain (Pimlott 1989; Jones and Kandiah 1996), it is possible to put forward a number of factors in support of this thesis. For instance, the succession of White Papers and reports emanating from the wartime coalition government highlighted the way in which cross-party concords could be secured in areas such as education, health, employment and social security. Indeed, in three key areas of reform – education, social security and health – the guiding lights were respectively Conservative (Butler), Liberal (Beveridge) and Labour (Bevan). Moreover, the influence of Keynes in the economic sphere (Williams and Williams 1995) –

which was evidenced in Kingsley Wood's budget of 1941 – and Beveridge (Silburn 1995) in the social sphere provided an opportunity to secure what Lowe (1994: 43) has termed 'the constructive complementarity of economic and social policy'.

Although there were some similarities in the post-1945 welfare policies pursued by both major parties in government, it is questionable whether this can accurately be described as a fully fledged consensus (Deakin 1994). Undoubtedly there was a degree of cross-party support for a mixed economy, high levels of employment and a mature welfare state. However, the existence of fundamental policy differences over such key issues as equality, redistribution and universalism suggests that any accord was of a shallow rather than a deep kind.

How then did young single mothers fare during this era? In general one could argue that there was a modest improvement in the position of this group during this period. First, it was accepted that the state should meet the subsistence needs of single mothers who had inadequate resources. Although excluded from Beveridge's social insurance scheme, young single mothers (like 'less deserving' separated and divorced mothers) were granted the right to claim means-tested social security benefits – a policy which provided them with an opportunity to secure an 'independent' existence, albeit of an impoverished kind (Marsden 1973; Hopkinson 1976). The inadequacy of support for this group led the Labour government to set up the Finer Committee on one-parent families in 1969. Its Report, which was published in 1974, provided a comprehensive review of social-security support for this group as well as a detailed discussion of the structure and effect of family law and maintenance procedures. The expectation that the Committee's policy recommendations would be 'practical', economically viable and fair (the maintenance of equity between one- and two-parent families was stressed) clearly limited the possibility of radical reform. Nevertheless, a determined attempt was made to improve the economic and social security of single parents, not least by the recommended introduction of a 'Guaranteed Maintenance Allowance'. The reluctance of the then Labour government to act on this proposal inevitably resulted in continued reliance on means-tested benefits for substantial numbers of lone parents. However, the special needs of lone-parent claimants had been acknowledged by the introduction of a small additional allowance (one-parent premium) and the introduction of more liberal eligibility rules (mothers were not required to under-take paid work or to disclose the identity of the 'absent' father).

Other advances in the treatment of single mothers are also worthy of note. In the field of housing there was a gradual accept-ance that lone parents should be entitled to accommodation on the same basis as two-parent families. By the end of the 1960s many Local Authorities dispensed with allocation procedures which discriminated against lone-parent families – a process which was strengthened following the introduction of the 1977 Housing (Homeless Persons) Act. Under this, Local Authorities were obliged to take responsibility for all those who were deemed to be non-intentionally homeless and in acute need. Local-authority housing has become the main form of tenure for lone parents (60 per cent). Although far from luxurious, council housing has provided the single mother with a reasonably secure, affordable home which is clearly an improvement on either hostel or shared accommodation.

The availability of financial support and accommodation has enabled young single mothers to resist the pressures to place their child for adoption, as has the development of a less judgmental form of social work. More generally, single mothers have benefited from what Lewis (1992) describes as the deregulation of private life. In an era in which divorce, abortion and homosexuality were more readily accepted, it was inevitable that greater tolerance would also be shown to single mothers. Indeed the decision by the National Council for the Unmarried Mother and her Child to change its title to the National Council for One Parent Families in 1969 was indicative of a desire to emphasis the similarity, rather than the diversity, of the lone-parent experience – an approach which also underpinned the attempt to standardise the legal position of illegitimate and legiti-mate citizens, in The Family Law Reform Act of 1969 and The Inheritance (Family and Dependants) Act of 1975 (Macaskill 1993).

Back to the margins? The New Right challenge to single motherhood

One of the reasons why 'traditional' social administration (Wilding 1983) has been subjected to critical appraisal in the recent past has been its rather too ready acceptance of what Baker (1979) has termed 'the social conscience' thesis. From this perspective, progres-sive ideas gradually come to the fore, with the result that contemporary public attitudes and levels of welfare provision come to be regarded as the most 'progressive' and 'humane' yet devised.

Type of one-parent family with dependent children	Numbers (thousands)									Average annual percentage increase in numbers	
	1971	1976	1986	1987	1988	1989	1990	1991	1992*	1971–86	1987–92*
Lone fathers	70	90	100	100	100	100	110	100	120	+3	+4
Lone mothers	500	660	910	960	980	1,060	1,120	1,200	1,280	+5	+7
Single	90	130	230	270	320	360	390	440	490	+10	+16
Separated	170	185	190	200	200	230	240	260	300	+1	+10
Divorced	120	230	410	410	390	400	420	430	430	+16	+1
Widowed	120	115	80	70	70	70	70	70	60	-2	-3
All one-parent families with dependent children	570	750	1,010	1,050	1,090	1,160	1,230	1,300	1,400	+5	+7

Table 8.1   Estimates of the number of one-parent families with dependent children, by type – Great Britain, 1971–92

Source: Haskey (1996), table 4, p. 11
Note: * provisional estimates

While this thesis does indeed need to be treated with caution it would appear to have some validity in the case of single mothers. The economic and social situation of this group has improved over the centuries. By the mid-1970s single mothers were no longer subject to public forms of humiliation of a religious or secular kind. They were not subjected to physical punishments, punitive forms of midwifery, or confinement to a penitentiary, workhouse, mother-and-baby home or mental hospital, nor were they cruelly pressurised to relinquish their child for adoption (Page 1984). However, the limitations of the social conscience thesis have been brought into sharp focus in the more recent past.

The return to power in 1979 of a Conservative government, with its clear commitment to move away from the post-1945 welfare 'consensus', should have sounded a warning to those who had come to believe in the inevitability of progress. By the 1990s lone parenthood had returned towards the top of the political agenda, not because of some urgent desire to improve the position of this group but, rather, to contain its growth and its seemingly voracious appetite for public funds. In essence, lone-parent families were once again being seen as a problem *for*, rather than an integral part *of*, society. In examining this issue it is useful, first to look at current trends in single motherhood.

TRENDS IN SINGLE MOTHERHOOD

There has been a significant growth in the number of single mothers over the past 25 years. Although single mothers still represent a minority of all lone-parent families, they now account for 35 per cent (490,000) of this group (1992) compared to 16 per cent in 1971 (90,000) (see Table 8.1). Single women are now the largest sub-group of lone mothers, whereas in 1971 they were the smallest. The growth in cohabitation is likely to be one reason for this increase (i.e. the single-mother category will have been swollen by former cohabiters – see Burghes with Brown 1995; L. Clarke 1996).

Forty-six per cent of contemporary single mothers are under 25, compared to around 5 per cent of other lone mothers (see Table 8.2). They make up 7.3 per cent of all families with dependent children. Single-mother families tend to be smaller (1.4 children per family) than either other lone-parent (1.7 children per family, on average) or two-parent families (1.9 children per family). However, the size of single-mother families is increasing (1.2 children per

	Single lone mother	Other lone mother	Cohabiting couples	Married couples
	%	%	%	%
Up to 20	8.6	0.3	2.8	0.2
20–24	37.4	4.5	21.3	4.5
25 and over	54.0	95.3	75.8	95.3

Table 8.2   Current age of mother – proportions by age group
Source: Burghes with Brown (1995), table 3, p. 21

family in 1981) – a trend which can be explained in part by an increase in the median age of this sub-group (Haskey 1994).

In discussions about young single mothers a distinction is often drawn between teenage mothers and those in their early twenties. While both groups are biologically mature (the age of menarche is around 13), it is often suggested that teenage mothers, unlike their older counterparts, are socially immature (Phoenix 1991). Phoenix acknowledges that very young mothers are likely to be socially immature.

> Most people would agree that at 14 years or less, young women in industrialised societies are not socially prepared for mother-hood. They are not legally allowed to leave full time education, to have sexual intercourse, to marry or enter into certain financial arrangements.
>
> (Phoenix 1991: 4)

However, she is equally clear 'that while mothers who are in their teenage years are clearly young people, most are not "young mothers". That is to say, they are not too young to be adequate mothers.' (ibid.: 4). Importantly, it should be noted that the number of conceptions to very young single women (under 15s) is relatively small: 7,243 conceptions in 1993 – 48.8 per cent of which were not carried to term (Office for National Statistics 1996).

As Table 8.3 indicates, the highest number of teenage births occurred in 1966 (86,746), although only 26 per cent of these were born out of wedlock. By 1976 this proportion had risen to 34 per cent (though the total number of births had declined), and by 1992 the vast majority of teenage births were to unmarried women (83.7 per cent). It is now much more common for extra-marital births of this kind to be jointly registered. In 1976 two-thirds of these births were sole

Year	Total births	Rate[1]	Births outside marriage	Rate[2]	Proportion[3] outside marriage
1951	29,111	21.3	4,812	3.7	165
1956	37,938	27.3	6,290	4.8	166
1961	59,786	37.3	11,896	8.0	199
1966	86,746	47.9	20,582	12.2	237
1971	82,641	50.6	21,555	14.6	261
1976	57,943	32.2	19,819	11.9	342
1981	56,570	28.1	26,430	13.2	406
1983	54,059	26.9	30,423	19.7	648
1986	57,406	30.1	39,613	21.3	690
1988	58,741	32.4	44,642	25.3	760
1990	55,541	33.3	44,583	27.4	802
1991	52,396	33.1	43,448	28.0	829
1992	47,900	31.8	40,100		837

Table 8.3   Live births to women under 20 – 1951–92
Source: Selman and Glendinning (1996), table 14.1, p. 204
Notes:
[1] per 1,000 women aged 15–19
[2] per 1,000 single, widowed or divorced women aged 15–19
[3] per 1,000 live births

registrations (64 per cent sole, 36 per cent joint), but by 1991 joint registrations had become much more commonplace (35 per cent sole, 65 per cent joint – see Table 8.4). Moreover, as Selman and Glendinning (1996: 205) remark, 'in a majority of these joint registrations both parents gave the same address, implying a degree of stability and even cohabitation, at least around the time of the child's birth.' The incidence of young single motherhood has also been affected by three other factors. Nearly a third of all teenage conceptions are terminated, although this does vary by region (44 per cent in the south-east, 27 per cent in the north – Selman and Glendinning, 1996: 207). Moreover, the number of 'unwed conceptions' subsequently legitimated by marriage has dropped sharply. Finally, far

Year	Total Births	Registration		(Joint registration) Address	
		Sole	Joint	Different	Same
		%	%	%	%
1964	17,400	81	19		
1971	21,555	72	28		
1976	19,819	64	36		
1981	26,430	52	48		
1986	39,613	41	59	[26]	[33]
1991	43,448	35	65	[27]	[38]

Table 8.4   Extra-marital teenage births (by registration)
Source: Selman and Glendinning (1996), table 14.2, p. 205

fewer children (especially very young infants) are now placed for adoption (8,000 in 1992 compared to a peak of 27,000 in 1968).

The vast majority of single mothers are dependent on Income Support. In 1993, 464,000 single mothers (47 per cent of all lone-parent claimants) and their children (726,000) were dependent on Income Support. The majority of these claimants (371,000) were between the ages of 20 and 34 (38,000 were aged 16–19). Some 228,000 lone parents were also in receipt of Family Credit in 1994, but single mothers were not major claimants of this benefit (Department of Social Security 1994). The growing dependence of single mothers on Income Support has coincided with a decline in the numbers engaged in part-time or full-time work; it has been estimated that in 1990–92 some 29 per cent of single mothers were economically active, compared to 49 per cent of other lone mothers and 63 of married mothers (see Table 8.5). Crucially, there appears to be a marked decline in the labour-market participation of lone mothers (especially among those caring for a child under 5); the converse is the case for married mothers.

The former Conservative government's desire to reduce public-spending commitments inevitably led to an ongoing review of social-security expenditure, which is forecast to rise beyond the £100 billion mark by the turn of the century. Given that the budget for lone parenthood is effectively open-ended, it is understandable

	Single lone mother	Other lone mother	Cohabiting couples	Married couples
	%	%	%	%
Working	28.7	49.1	53.7	63.5
Seeking work	7.5	5.1	5.7	3.0
Keeping house	60.5	40.4	38.8	31.7
Other/inactive	3.3	5.3	1.8	1.8

Table 8.5   Economic activity of mothers, 1990–92
Source: Burghes with Brown (1995), table 9, p. 23

that an administration seeking to preserve its reputation for reducing state activity will endeavour to curb the growth of this form of dependence (total spending on lone parents was £9.4 billion in 1995/6).

PARENTAL DEFICIENCIES

The social viability of the single-mother household has also been brought into question. Undoubtedly, the commentator who has been most influential in identifying the single mother – as opposed to lone parents in general – as a problem for society is Charles Murray (1984,1990,1994). As he states 'one particular form of single parenthood – illegitimacy – constitutes a special problem for society. Single parent families are radically unequal' (Murray 1990: 8). Murray contends that the recent growth in single motherhood can be linked to the increased generosity of the welfare system, for example higher benefits and access to Local-Authority accommodation. For Murray, provision of this kind provides unwarranted opportunities for young single women from the lowest social classes to raise a family at public expense. Given their limited schooling, these women are, according to Murray, much more likely than other lone parents to become long-term dependants on social assistance.

The growth in the number of 'independent' single-mother households concerns Murray. He believes that the children from such families will be inappropriately socialised, not least because they will tend to live in neighbourhoods in which two-parent families are in a minority. In particular, young mothers will find it difficult to socialise boys or find appropriate role models for them in their local community. The result, according to Murray, is clear: the growth of the underclass.

> The key to an underclass is not the individual instance but a situation in which a very large proportion of an entire community lacks fathers, and this is far more common in poor communities than in rich ones.
>
> (Murray 1990: 13)

For Murray, then, the growth of young single motherhood could be said to increase, rather than reduce, class divisions in society.

It is not just those on the right of the political spectrum who have expressed concern about the social impact of lone motherhood. Both Norman Dennis (Dennis and Erdos 1992) and Frank Field (1995), writing from an ethical socialist standpoint, have expressed concern about the growth of poorly functioning families and the increased levels of adult selfishness and irresponsibility (particularly among younger men). Like Murray, Dennis and Erdos believe that families in which the natural father is present rather than absent will function far more effectively: 'The longer the same father has been part of the child's life, and the more effectively the father has taken part in the life of the family, the better the results for the child' (Dennis and Erdos: 1992: 44).

Frank Field (1995) has also voiced his concern about single mothers, as opposed to other forms of lone parenthood. While he accepts that some degree of marital breakdown is inevitable (ibid.: 11), he regards the growth of 'very young single mothers' as more problematic. According to Field these mothers are likely to be 'the least able of their peer group' with the 'fewest basic skills and low levels of literacy' (ibid.: 42). Children living in such households are not only likely to have a financially impoverished existence but also a socially deprived one.

> imagine what it is like never to have known one's father. What does it mean for hundreds of thousands and possibly, by now, millions of young people that their mother has had a number of other partners, most of whom gave her children – their step-brothers and sisters? What message is being put across to

children when much of family life is spent eating in front of a TV screen while a succession of different boyfriends occupy the seats behind them?

(Field 1995: 13)

Is there any evidence to support the assertion that the children of single mothers will be economically and socially disadvantaged? The 'viability' or otherwise of the lone-parent family has been the subject of a good deal of research in the post-war period (see reviews by Page 1984; Burghes 1994, 1996). Much of this research relates to all forms of lone parenthood, rather than simply single mothers. There would appear to be little dispute that dependent children living in lone-parent households are likely to be economically disadvantaged, to be in poorer health, to perform less well at school and to be over-represented in poorer-paid forms of employment during adulthood (Crellin *et al.* 1971; Hunt *et al.* 1973; Ferri 1976; Gill 1977; Lambert and Streather 1980; Ferri (ed.) 1993). There is less unanimity on such issues as whether children from lone-parent families suffer long-term emotional damage (Burghes 1994, 1996) or are more prone to criminality (Utting *et al.* 1993).

Part of the problem in resolving this issue is the difficulty of obtaining 'conclusive' evidence. For example, it can be argued that the disadvantages of contemporary adults who grew up in a lone-parent household during the 1950s or 1960s (which are captured by longitudinal studies – see Crellin *et al.* 1971; Ferri (ed.) 1993; Spence *et al.* 1954; Kolvin *et al.* 1992) should not form the basis for contemporary policy initiatives, given that their experiences are likely to be significantly different from those children currently living in a lone-parent family (Burghes 1994). It is also possible that the negative aspects of lone parenthood have been exaggerated by the selective reporting of the behaviour and achievements of 'lone-parent' children by 'gatekeepers', such as teachers, doctors, social workers and the police. Moreover, it is important to remember that many children only live in lone-parent households for *part* of their childhood (Millar 1989).

Roseneil and Mann (1996) also contend that the recent attacks on single mothers should be seen as part of a concerted anti-feminist backlash. They argue that the modest gains which women have achieved in their struggle to secure economic and social independence from men is now leading to determined efforts to re-establish patriarchal structures, by the reaffirmation of the virtues of the heterosexual nuclear family, by the emphasis given to good 'mothering' and by the increasing focus on the plight of men, not least because of their growing vulnerability to unemployment.

THE POLICY RESPONSE TO YOUNG SINGLE MOTHERS: REDUCING STATE DEPENDENCE

Social security

As noted above, recent Conservative governments have been keen to stem the rise in the social security budget. This has led to policy initiatives designed to reduce the level of dependence among lone parents. For example, modest attempts have been made to improve the financial situation of lone parents who wish to return to work by bolstering the Family Credit scheme – which recent evidence tends to suggest can play a part in improving the labour-market participation of lone parents (Marsh and McKay 1993; McKay and Marsh 1994) – and by providing some assistance with child-care costs. In addition, a Child Support Agency has been created following the publication of the White Paper *Children Come First* in 1990. This agency, which has been operating since April 1993, has been charged with the responsibility of collecting realistic forms of maintenance from absent parents. It is envisaged that awards to mothers with care will provide a financial platform for them to return to the labour market. As has been widely reported, the Agency has encountered a number of major difficulties and has been heavily criticised on a number of grounds: its rigid assessment formula, which fails to acknowledge the diverse financial circumstances of liable relatives; its failure to recognise the position of second families; the absence of a satisfactory appeals procedure; the lack of appropriate 'co-operative incentives' (e.g. ensuring that payments from absent parents enhance the well-being of dependants, rather than the Treasury – Millar and Whiteford 1993); the targeting of 'good payers' rather than non-payers; punitive sanctions for non-cooperative parents with care; and poor administrative and assessment procedures.

Crucially, the argument put forward by commentators such as Morgan (1995), that lone parents are treated more favourably by the social-security system than two-parent families, has now been firmly accepted in Conservative circles, despite continuing evidence which confirms that lone parents incur higher living costs than their two-parent counterparts (Kempson 1996). In the 1995 Budget the lone-parent premium payable under the Income Support scheme was frozen, as was one-parent benefit. It is possible that both these benefits will eventually be phased out.

Housing

Lone parents' entitlement to publicly rented housing has also been weakened (Department of the Environment 1994a, 1994b, 1995). In particular, Local Authorities are now only required to provide 'accommodation for a limited period for applicants who are in priority need, in an immediate crisis that has arisen through no fault of their own' and who, moreover, 'have no alternative accommodation available to which they could reasonably be expected to go' (Department of the Environment 1994a: para. 3.2). This would appear to signal a return to the less eligible ethos of the not-so-distant past (Pascall and Morley 1996). Indeed, the whole thrust of Conservative policy in this area has been to encourage responsible parenting (i.e. economically independent two-parent households) by the removal of fast-track entry into Local-Authority housing for young single mothers. The Conservatives envisage that this policy shift will discourage single motherhood by reinforcing the importance of planned and stable parenthood.

Although it is clear that the homelessness legislation has, as intended, given priority to the housing needs of parents with dependent children (both married and unmarried), there is little systematic evidence to suggest that significant numbers of young single women have opted for motherhood in order to obtain permanent accommodation, despite ministerial and other protestations to the contrary (for example, by Peter Lilley in October 1992, Sir George Young in October 1993 and John Redwood in August 1995). Indeed the idea that there might be some general validity in this suggestion has been vigorously contested – not least when it was advanced in a controversial edition of the BBC current-affairs programme *Panorama*, 'Babies on Benefit' (see Broadcasting Complaints Commission 1994).

Adoption

One leading Conservative thinker – John Redwood (1995) – has also voiced his concern about whether young single mothers should be permitted to subsist on social security. If a young mother is unable to obtain financial support from the father of her child or members of her extended family, Redwood contends that adoption would be a better solution than 'a life of premature motherhood and domesticity, married to the State and dependent on benefit.' The idea that young mothers might be encouraged to opt for adoption is echoed in recent Conservative proposals for reform in this area. While the new legislation might have some advantages, the fact that it permits children to be adopted against the expressed wish of their natural parents (Department of Health 1996) remains a cause for concern. Redwood also suggests that those young mothers who opt for state support should be provided with a hostel place which enables them to work and study, rather than Income Support and a council flat of their own.

Reintroduction of stigma

More generally, it is clear that there is support in Conservative circles for the reintroduction of stigma as a means of reducing the incidence of single motherhood. As Digby Anderson (1995) comments: '[stigma] is the obverse of approval. No society has ever done without it. Once this is admitted, one can concentrate on the important task of focusing the stigma appropriately, so that it sustains rather than subverts respectable families.'

TOWARDS CLASSLESSNESS? IS THERE A WAY FORWARD?

The notion of classlessness favoured by John Major should not be equated with any heartfelt desire to bring about a society in which social and economic divisions wither away. Like other Conservatives of varying hues, Major favours an unequal society, but is keen to ensure that the differences which emerge are perceived to be legitimate – i.e. based on genuine variations in skills and abilities. In essence, this requires a commitment to equality of opportunity. There must be no artificial barriers to taking one's rightful place in society. Even if one accepts this limited notion of classlessness, it is clear that a number of social-policy initiatives will be needed if young single mothers are to become fully integrated members of society with opportunities for economic and social advancement.

Education and training

As was noted earlier, young single mothers tend to come from poorer social-class backgrounds (Haskey 1996). They also tend to be less well educated and trained than their childless or married peers. Early parenthood often leads to interrupted schooling (Schofield 1995) or the curtailment of training, with the inevitable result that even those fortunate enough to secure entry into the labour market are rarely able to obtain well-paid work. Clearly, young mothers must be encouraged to stay on in full-time education in order to equip themselves with as wide a range of skills as possible in order to maximise their future life chances, not least in the labour market. Certainly, the Commission on Social Justice was persuaded of the merits of a Jobs, Education and Training programme (JET).

> The JET programme should transform the Employment Service into a 'one-stop re-employment shop' to advise the long-term unemployed about education and training services, career possibilities, job openings and child-care facilities, as well as help in moving from out-of-work to in-work benefits.
>
> (Commission on Social Justice 1994: 173)

However, even well-educated or well-trained single mothers are likely to experience difficulties when they attempt to enter the labour market, unless they can find affordable substitute care or supportive employers who will permit them to take time off work to fulfil care commitments.

Child care

The lack of affordable and available child-care facilities for pre-school children, as well as after school and holiday provision for older children, has been identified as a major barrier to the labour-market participation of single mothers. In part, the lack of such provision reflects continuing uncertainty about whether mothers, particularly those with young children, should be encouraged to enter the labour market or to stay at home (at least until their child reaches the age of five). Even if it is accepted that single mothers should become financially independent, questions remain about the relative responsibilities of Government, employers or mothers in terms of arranging or financing substitute care

(Morgan 1996). Clearly an expansion of state provision in this area would be advantageous, although it is unlikely to be a favoured policy option as far as the current Conservatives are concerned, given their belief that the role of the state should be limited to that of facilitator rather than provider or sole financier. This approach to child care has been bolstered by survey evidence which suggests that lone parents are able to make informal care arrangements (Marsh and McKay 1993). Although the Labour Party believes that a more proactive approach to child care is required, its current predilection for fiscal rectitude is unlikely to lead to dramatic improvements in this area.

Employment opportunities

If young single mothers are expected to finance substitute care in whole or in part from their own earnings, they will obviously need to be able to find relatively well-paid work. Even though women are entering the labour force in ever increasing numbers, they are not tending to command the kinds of rewards which make paid work a viable option. Although the Conservatives have proved willing to top up low pay through Family Credit, it is clear that single mothers will continue to be prone to poverty even if they manage to obtain paid work. Moreover, even if Labour's more ambitious plans for education and training are brought into effect, there is no guarantee that Britain will be able to command an increased share of well-paid employment, given the highly competitive nature of the global economic environment in which corporate and shareholder interests have now transcended any loyalty to the nation state (Held 1995; Hirst and Thompson 1996).

Housing

In order to become full members of society, single mothers must be able to acquire affordable, self-contained housing (Speak *et al.* 1995). Given that this group, like all low-paid workers, finds it difficult to gain entry into the owner-occupied sector, it is imperative that a good supply of affordable Local-Authority or Housing-Association accommodation is made available. The pursuit of this objective will not only necessitate a re-appraisal of the decision to move away from the public provision of rented housing, and a reversal of those measures which have weakened lone parents' eligibility for such accommodation, but also a return to affordable rent levels. Although the decision in the 1996 Budget to limit young people's entitlement to housing benefit does not affect the single-mother group at present, it is possible that it may be targeted in the future.

Financial support

Since the rejection of Finer's Guaranteed Maintenance Allowance in the 1970s the idea of providing adequate state allowances for parents who care for their children on a full-time basis has not been given serious consideration. Again, there are a number of reasons for this. First, it is contended that a benefit solely designed for lone parents would create inequities with regard to two-parent families. Second, the issue of whether single mothers should be permitted to become full-time carers remains a contentious one. For example, some feminists believe that support of this kind reinforces gendered patterns of care and fails to challenge occupational segregation, inflexible workplace practices and resource inequalities; as such, it should be regarded as an example of state patriarchy (Walby 1990). Others focus on the long-term disadvantage that can accrue to women who remain out of the labour market for lengthy periods of time. For example, the Commission on Social Justice (1994) has suggested that all lone parents whose youngest child reaches the age of five should, unless there are pressing reasons to the contrary, be 'required' to undertake paid work rather than remain at home. This denial of a carer's option is justified on the grounds that it will be to the long-term advantage of the mothers concerned.

While the disadvantages of home care allowances should not be minimised, it is equally important not to over-romanticise the world of paid work. For the vast majority of lone mothers, labour market participation does not provide an opportunity for breaking through glass ceilings but, rather, for being nailed, almost literally, to unpolished floors. Clearly an adequate carer's allowance scheme is likely to prove a far more attractive option (Thomson 1995) than trying to combine child-care responsibilities with soul-destroying low-paid work. Although the advocacy of a carer's allowance might sound like a return to the world of Hobhouse and Beveridge, it has some undoubted strengths, not least the opportunity it affords for making meaningful choices with regard to care and work packages. In conjunction with effective education and training programmes, generous end-of-parenting allowances and guaranteed pension rights, a policy of this kind could help to promote classlessness. Again, though, the thrust of contemporary Conservative policy is to deny claimants the right to subsist on benefits for lengthy periods of time, as witnessed by the introduction of a pilot workfare scheme (Project Work) in Hull and Kent and the implementation of the Jobseekers Allowance scheme in the autumn of 1996.

Even if the economic situation of young single mothers improves, it is still questionable whether they will achieve full social acceptance. In the current climate it seems unlikely that there will be a ground swell of public support for the pursuit of what can be termed 'reactive', as opposed to 'proactive', forms of family policy. From a 'reactive' perspective, decisions about family formations should be regarded as a private matter for individual resolution. If more young women wish to bring up children without a father, then the task of social policy should be to ensure that supportive structures are in place which enable them to live full and satisfying lives. This would mean that the state would assume responsibility for the provision of appropriate material resources and for adjudicating in cases where there is a 'legitimate' dispute between parents (e.g. over care or access arrangements). However, those who believe that it is important to construct policies which reinforce a particular type of family formation (heterosexual couples with children) are likely to favour intervention of a more 'proactive' kind. This may involve the construction of welfare packages which provide distinctive advantages to two-parent, as opposed to lone-parent, households and the reaffirmation of parents' obligations towards their children.

CONCLUSION

It has proved notoriously difficult to construct social policies for single mothers and the lone-parent family group more generally because of the existence of a number of competing objectives. As Bradshaw (1989) notes, attempts to improve the living standards and rights of lone mothers (basic living standard, training and work opportunities and the establishment of the right to opt out of labour market participation) often conflict with other objectives (a desire to reduce dependence on benefits, the discouragement of marital breakdown and illegitimacy, ensuring absent parents make appropriate contributions to their children and an unwillingness to leave lone-parent families better off than two-parent families). Although a number of commentators have drawn attention to the

difficulties in attempting to counter emerging trends in family formation (Ermisch 1991; Kiernan and Estaugh 1993; Burghes 1993;
Hewitt and Leach 1993), proactive forms of social policy would
appear to be in the ascendancy with regard to the treatment of young
single mothers in Britain. It is premature to suggest that this will lead
to a situation in which British policy mirrors the more draconian
measures which are being piloted in some American states, such as
New Jersey, where additional benefits are being denied to single
mothers who increase the size of their family while on 'welfare'.
However, it seems clear that the rights of single mothers in Britain to
claim public assistance will depend more on demonstrations of
personal responsibility, such as the compilation of return-to-work
plans (Field 1995: 188), not least because of this group's limited
popularity with the general public (Taylor-Gooby 1987, 1991). Those
mothers who are unable or unwilling to make stringent efforts to end
their dependence on state support, even in the absence of comprehensive substitute care provision, are likely to find themselves
subjected to more stringent forms of social control. Crucially, it
appears that one of the main aims of current welfare initiatives is to
ensure that the lone-parent group is fragmented, so that more punitive measures can be directed towards young single mothers. In a
climate of this kind classlessness would appear to be a distant dream,
not just for today's single mothers but for those yet to come.

REFERENCES

Anderson, D. (1995) 'Illegitimacy *should* be shameful', *The Times*, 15
    August 1996.
Anstruther, I. (1973) *The Scandal of the Andover Workhouse*, London:
    Geoffrey Bles.
Baker, J. (1979) 'Social conscience and social policy', *Journal of Social
    Policy* 8(2): 177–206.
Bowlby, J. (1965) *Child Care and the Growth of Love*, 2nd ed.,
    Harmondsworth: Penguin.
Bradshaw, J. (1989) *Lone Parents: Policy in the Doldrums*, London: Family
    Policy Studies Centre.
Broadcasting Complaints Commission (1994) *Complaint from National
    Council for One Parent Families*, London: BCC.
Burghes, L. (1993) *One-Parent Families: Policy Options for the 1990s*, York:
    Joseph Rowntree Foundation.
—— (1994) *Lone Parenthood and Family Disruption: The Outcomes for
    Children*, Occasional Paper No. 18, London: Family Policy Studies
    Centre.
—— (1996) 'Debates on disruption: What happens to the children of lone

parents' in E. B. Silva (ed.) *Good Enough Mothering*, London: Routledge.

Burghes, L. with Brown, M. (1995) *Single Lone Mothers: Problems, Prospects and Policies*, London: Family Policy Studies Centre.

Cheetham, J. (1977) *Unwanted Pregnancy and Counselling*, London: Routledge & Kegan Paul.

Children Come First (1990), CM 1264, London: HMSO.

Clarke, L. (1996) 'Demographic change and the family situation of children', in J. Brannen and M. O'Brien (eds) *Children in Families*, London: Falmer.

Clarke, P. (1996) *Hope and Glory*, London: Allen Lane.

Commission on Social Justice (1994) *Social Justice: Strategies for National Renewal*, London: Vintage.

Crellin, E., Kellmer Pringle, M.L. and West, P. (1971) *Born Illegitimate*, Windsor: National Council for Educational Research in England and Wales.

Deakin, N. (1994) *The Politics of Welfare*, Hemel Hempstead: Harvester Wheatsheaf.

Dennis, N. and Erdos, G. (1992) *Families Without Fatherhood*, London: IEA.

Department of the Environment (1994a) *Access to Local Authority and Housing Association Tenancies: A Consultation Paper*, London: DOE.

—— (1994b) *Access to Local Authority and Housing Association Tenancies: Main Changes Proposed to the Present Homelessness Legislation in Light of the January 1994 Consultation Paper*, London: DOE.

—— (1995) *Our Future Homes: Opportunity, Choice Responsibility*, London: HMSO.

Department of Health (1996) *Adoption – A Service for Children*, London: Department of Health.

Department of Social Security, (1994) *Social Security Statistics 1994*, London: HMSO.

Dutton, D. (1991) *British Politics Since 1945: The Rise and Fall of Consensus*, Oxford: Blackwell.

Emmison, F.G. (1973) *Elizabethan Life: Morals and the Church Courts*, Chelmsford: Essex County Council.

Ermisch, J.F. (1991) *Lone Parenthood: An Economic Analysis*, NIESR Research Paper No. XLIV., Cambridge: Cambridge University Press.

Eysenck, S.B.G. (1961) 'Personality and pain assessment in childbirth of married and unmarried mothers', *British Journal of Mental Science* 107: 417–30.

Ferguson, S.M. and Fitzgerald, H. (1954) *Studies in the Social Services*, London: HMSO and Longmans, Green & Co.

Ferri, E. (1976), *Growing Up in a One-Parent Family*, Windsor: National Council for Educational Research in England and Wales.

—— (ed.), (1993) *Britain's 33 Year Olds – The Fifth Follow-Up to the National Child Development Study*, London: NCH/ESRC.

Field, F. (1995) *Making Welfare Work: Reconstructing Welfare for the Millennium*, London: Institute of Community Studies.

Finer Report (1974), *Report of the Committee on One-Parent Families* Vol. 1, Cmnd 5629, London: HMSO.

Finlayson, G. (1994) *Citizen, State and Social Welfare in Britain 1830–1990*, Oxford: Clarendon Press.

Floyd, J. and Viney, L.L. (1974) 'Ego identity and ego ideal in the unwed mother', *British Journal of Medical Psychology* 47: 273–81.

Gill, D. (1977) *Illegitimacy, Sexuality and the State*, Oxford: Blackwell.

Greenberg, N.G. *et al.* (1959) 'Life situations associated with the onset of pregnancy', *Psychosomatic Medicine* 31(4): 296–310.

Hair, P.E.H. (1966) 'Bridal pregnancy in rural England in earlier centuries', *Population Studies* 20(2), November: 233–43.

—— (1970) 'Bridal pregnancy in earlier rural England further examined', *Population Studies* 24(1), March: 59–70.

Haskey, J. (1994) 'Estimated numbers of one-parent families and their prevalence in Great Britain in 1991', *Population Trends*, 78, Winter: 5–19.

—— (1996) 'Population review: (6) families and households in Great Britain', *Population Trends* 85, Autumn: 7–24.

Held, D. (1995) *Democracy and the Global Order*, Cambridge: Polity Press.

Helmholz, R.M. (1975) 'Infanticide in the province of Canterbury during the fifteenth century', *History of Childhood Quarterly* 2: 379–90.

Hewitt, P. and Leach, P. (1993) *Social Justice, Children and Families*, London: IPPR.

Heywood, J. (1978) *Children in English Society*, London: Routledge & Kegan Paul.

Hirst, P. and Thompson, G. (1996) *Globalization in Question*, Cambridge: Polity Press

Hopkinson, A, (1976) *Single Mothers: The First Year*, Edinburgh: Scottish Council for Single Parents.

Hunt, A., Fox, J. and Morgan, M. (1973) *Families and Their Needs with Particular Reference to One-Parent Families*, OPCS Survey Div., Vol. 1, London: HMSO.

Jones, H. and Kandiah, M. (eds) (1996) *The Myth of Consensus*, London: Macmillan.

Kempson, E. (1996) *Life on a Low Income*, York: Joseph Rowntree Foundation.

Kiernan, K.E. and Estaugh, V. (1993) *Cohabitation: Extra-Marital Childbearing and Social Policy*, Occasional Paper No. 17, London: Family Policy Studies Centre.

Kolvin, I., Miller, F.J.W., Scott, D. McL., Gatzanis, S.R.M. and Fleeting, M., (1992) *Continuities In Deprivation?: The Newcastle 1000 Family Study*, Aldershot: Avebury.

Lambert, L. and Streather, J. (1980) *Children in Changing Families*, London: Macmillan.

Laslett, P., Oosterveen, K. and Smith, R.M. (eds) (1980) *Bastardy and Its Comparative History*, London: Edward Arnold.

Lewis, J. (1992) *Women in Britain Since 1945*, Oxford: Blackwell.

Longmate, N. (1974) *The Workhouse*, London: Temple Smith.

Lowe, R. (1990) 'The Second World War: Consensus and the foundation of the welfare state', *Twentieth Century British History* 1(2): 152–82.

—— (1994) 'Lessons from the past: The rise and fall of the classic welfare state in Britain, 1945–76', in A. Oakley and A.S. Williams (eds) *The Politics of the Welfare State*, UCL: London.

Macaskill, H. (1993) *From the Workhouse to the Workplace*, National Council for One Parent Families, London.

Macfarlane, A. (1980) 'Illegitimacy and illegitimacies in English history', in P. Laslett, K. Oosterveen and R.M. Smith (eds), *Bastardy and Its Comparative History*, London: Edward Arnold.

McKay, S. and Marsh, A. (1994) *Lone Parents and Work*, DSS Research Report No. 25, London: HMSO.

Macnicol, J. (1980) *The Movement for Family Allowances, 1918–45: A Study in Social Policy Development*, London: Heinemann.

Marks, L. (1992) ' "The luckless waifs and strays of humanity": Irish and Jewish immigrant unwed mothers in London, 1870–1939', *Twentieth Century British History*, 3(2): 113–37.

Marsden, D. (1973) *Mothers Alone*, Harmondsworth: Penguin.

Marsh, A. and McKay, S. (1993) *Families, Work and Benefits*, London: PSI.

May, G. (1930) *Social Control of Sex Expression*, London: George Allen & Unwin.

Middleton, N. (1971) *When Family Failed*, London: Victor Gollancz.

Millar, J. (1989) *Poverty and The Lone Parent Family: The Challenge To Social Policy,* Aldershot: Avebury.

Millar, J. and Whiteford, P. (1993) 'Child support in lone parent families: Policies in Australia and the UK', *Policy and Politics* 21(1): 59–72.

Morgan, P. (1995) *Farewell to the Family*, London: IEA.

—— (1996) 'Careless child', *Prospect*, October: 14–15.

Murray, C. (1984) *Losing Ground*, New York: Basic Books.

—— (1990) *The Emerging British Underclass*, London: IEA.

—— (1994) *Underclass: The Crisis Deepens*, London: IEA.

Naiman, J. (1966) 'A comparative study of unmarried and married mothers', *Canadian Psychiatric Association Journal* 11(6), December: 465–9.

—— (1971) 'A comparison between unmarried women seeking therapeutic abortion and unmarried mothers', *Laval Medicine* 42, December: 1086–8.

National Council for Civil Liberties (1951) *50,000 Outside the Law*, NCCL, London.

Office for National Statistics (1996) *1994 Birth Statistics*, London: HMSO.

Owen, D. (1965) *English Philanthropy, 1660–1960*, Massachusetts: Harvard University Press.

Oxley, G.W. (1974) *Poor Relief in England and Wales 1601–1834*, Newton Abbot: David & Charles.

Page, R.M. (1984) *Stigma*, London: Routledge & Kegan Paul.

Pascall, G. and Morley, R. (1996) 'Women and homelessness: Proposals from the Department of the Environment', *Journal of Social Welfare and Family Law* 18(2): 189–202.

Phoenix, A. (1991) *Young Mothers*, Cambridge: Polity Press.

Pimlott, B. (1989) 'Controversy: Is the "postwar consensus" a myth?', *Contemporary Record* 2(6), Summer: 12–14.

Pinchbeck, I. and Hewitt, M. (1973) *Children in English Society, vol. II*, London: Routledge & Kegan Paul.

Rathbone, E.F. (1924) *The Disinherited Family*, London: George Allen & Unwin.

Redwood, J. (1995) 'Single mothers: Should the state always play nanny?', *Mail on Sunday*, 13 August 1995.

Roseneil, S. and Mann, K. (1996) 'Unpalatable choices and inadequate families: Lone mothers and the underclass debate', in E.B. Silva (ed.) *Good Enough Mothering*, London: Routledge.

Schofield, G. (1995) *The Youngest Mothers*, Aldershot: Avebury.

Selman, P. and Glendinning, C. (1996) 'Teenage pregnancy: Do social policies make a difference?', in J. Brannen and M. O'Brien, (eds) *Children in Families*, London: Falmer.

Shorter, E. (1977) *The Making of the Modern Family*, Glasgow: Fontana.

Silburn, R. (1995) 'Beveridge' in V. George and R. Page (eds) *Modern Thinkers on Welfare*, Hemel Hempstead: Prentice Hall/Harvester Wheatsheaf.

Smart, C. (1996) 'Deconstructing motherhood', in E.B. Silva (ed.) *Good Enough Mothering*, London: Routledge.

Speak, S., Cameron, S., Woods, R. and Gilroy, R. (1995) *Young Single Mothers: Barriers to Independent Living*, London: Family Policy Studies Centre.

Spence, J.C., Walton, W.S., Miller, F.J.W. and Court, S.D.M., (1954) *A Thousand Families in Newcastle Upon Tyne*, London: Oxford University Press.

Spensky, M. (1992) 'Producers of illegitimacy: Homes for unmarried mothers in the 1950s', in C. Smart (ed.) *Regulating Womanhood*, London: Routledge.

Taylor-Gooby, P. (1987) 'Citizenship and welfare' in R. Jowell, S. Witherspoon and L. Brook (eds), *British Social Attitudes: The 1987 Report*, Aldershot: Gower.

—— (1991) 'Attachment to the welfare state', in R. Jowell, L. Brook and B. Taylor with G. Prior (eds) *British Social Attitudes: The 8th Report*, Aldershot: Dartmouth.

Thompson, B. (1956) 'Social study of illegitimate maternities', *British Journal of Preventative and Social Medicine* 10: 75–87.

Thomson, K. (1995) 'Working mothers: Choice or circumstance?', in R. Jowell, J. Curtice, A. Park, L. Brook and D. Ahrendt, with K. Thomson (eds) *British Social Attitudes: The 12th Report*, Aldershot: Dartmouth.

Utting, D., Bright, J. and Henricson, C. (1993) *Crime and the Family: Improving Child-Rearing and Preventing Delinquency*, Occasional Paper No. 16, London: Family Policy Studies Centre.

Vincent, J.A. (1978) *Illegitimacy*, unpublished Ph.D. thesis, University of Surrey.

Walby, S. (1990) *Theorizing Patriarchy*, Oxford: Blackwell.

Wilding, P. (1983) 'The evolution of social administration', in P. Bean and S. MacPherson (eds), *Approaches to Welfare*, London: Routledge & Kegan Paul.

Williams, K. and Williams, J. (1995) 'Keynes', in V. George and R. Page (eds) *Modern Thinkers on Welfare*, Hemel Hempstead: Prentice Hall/Harvester Wheatsheaf

Winnicott, D. (1957) *The Child, The Family and the Outside World*, Harmondsworth, Penguin.

Yelloly, M.A. (1965) 'Factors relating to an adoption decision by the mothers of illegitimate infants', *Sociological Review* 13(1), March: 5–14.

Young. L. (1954) *Out of Wedlock*, New York: McGraw-Hill.

Chapter 9

British social work and the classless society
The failure of a profession

Chris Jones

INTRODUCTION

Preoccupied and focused, as it is, on the lives of some of the most vulnerable and deprived people in British society, social work ought to be ideally placed to comment upon John Major's claims that we are moving towards a classless society. Not only is the vast majority of its clients drawn from some of the most deprived and vulnerable segments of the working classes, this has been the traditional and principal domain of social work activity since its inception with the Charity Organisation Society (COS) in 1869. Social workers are involved with poor people, whatever other welfare label they may carry –such as people with special needs, elderly or lone parents. This has always been so. Social workers have a location and history which enables them to comment with some experience on class dynamics, inequality and social polarisation. As two Canadian social-work academics noted, this is true for social workers throughout the world: 'Social work is a profession that operates in almost every society across the world; and every day hundreds or thousands of social workers in each of these societies are dealing with some aspect or manifestation of poverty' (Larochelle and Campfens 1992: 105).

Yet as an occupation, or even as a profession (social work has a contested status), British social work has been peculiarly silent over the past twenty years about the shifting patterns in social well-being and disadvantage, even though poverty has engulfed entire neighbourhoods and localities with its attendant corrosion of well-being and self respect (Campbell 1993). Indeed, as Peter Townsend argued, the growing divide between the rich and the poor – as the rich have become wealthier and the poor more impoverished – constitutes 'the biggest single change in British society, and it has many ramifications' (Townsend 1995: 145). Moreover, as the Children's Rights Development Unit observed, not only have many children suffered as a consequence of these changes, but Britain, along with the USA, is at the leading edge of polarising societies:

> It is evident then that not only are there very substantial numbers of children living in poverty but that the numbers have escalated rapidly in recent years. This pattern contrasts sharply with most other European countries where not only is there less child poverty, but there has been no rise in child poverty in the 1980s. A report produced for UNICEF in 1993 the Index of Social Health seeks to monitor, over a 20 year period, the social well-being of children in industrial countries through a set of international indicators relating to children's health, education, emotional stress and economic welfare. The report demonstrates that of the 10 countries studied, only in the UK and US did children end the period with lower levels of social health on every count than they started with. In the UK, charting progress on an index of 0–100, the score was 20 points lower than in 1970.
>
> (CRDU 1994: 71)

So much for a classless society.

Since the early 1980s the resources allocated to state social work in particular, and social-welfare agencies in general, have not only failed to match these growing needs but in many instances have been reduced. The consequences for both social service agencies and clients have been significant. As Tessa Jowell, the then chair of the Social Services Committee of the Association of Metropolitan Authorities, noted:

> The personal social services seem to be moving from a situation of providers of barely adequate services for the poor towards becoming underfunded, overstretched and in some cases over-whelmed services for the oppressed. When the majority of persons referred to the social services are unwaged, when they are becoming poorer, when their chance of decent housing is declining and where their access to jobs is much less, then it is no exaggeration to describe many users of social services as an oppressed class.
>
> (cited in Balloch and Hume 1985: vi)

Oppenheim in commenting upon the impact of such changes on state social work practice in an Inner London borough observed that, 'gatekeeping is no longer subtle; we lock the front doors and if needs be put on the answerphone. The effect is frustrating for consumers and workers; anger is seemingly more in evidence and so is desperation' (Oppenheim 1987: 10). Given that social work is for many clients an agency of last resort – contact with which can often entail a degree of humiliation in order to secure some extra resources – it is hardly surprising that there has been an increase in the antagonism between social workers and their clients as hardship has deepened and resources shrunk (see Jordan 1988: 202). Social workers are now more likely to experience physical assault in the course of their work than police officers (NALGO 1989). It has become increasingly dangerous work (Parton and Small 1989). Clients are becoming not only more impoverished and more desperate, but social workers are finding themselves administering ever tighter and stricter eligibility rules; it is an explosive context. As Baldock summarised: 'There is, even more than is usual, an unresolved crisis of role and a deep sense of frustration and overload as British social workers face the daily evidence of an increasingly unequal but relatively uncaring society' (Baldock 1989: 25).

This chapter seeks to explore this changed context of social work practice – a context which in the past twenty years has had no resonance with John Major's aspirations for a classless society at ease with itself. Rather, social work finds itself at the wrong end of an increasingly polarised and divided society. In so doing the chapter seeks to understand what I take to be one of the most pertinent failings of social work during this period, namely its general silence and lack of presence in drawing attention to the human and social consequences of this process of impoverishment and social division.

EXPECTATIONS

Some might argue that the silence of social work organisations about these harder and more brutalising times should come as no surprise. After all, social work, with its traditional emphasis on the individualisation of social problems, must be considered as essentially a conservative activity. Social work, at least in its principal forms, has long been constructed around a set of idealistic premises according to which explanations of disadvantage and its associated problems have been primarily located in the manners, values and

behaviours of the poor themselves. That is not to say that traditional social work has eschewed the impact of unemployment, low
wages or poor housing, health chances and education on the well-
being of its clients. Rather, these social and economic factors have
been taken as being of secondary importance when compared with
the character and outlook of clients. Social work has implicitly (and
at times explicitly) been developed within a social Darwinian
paradigm which implies that those at the bottom of the social
system are there by virtue of their impaired character (Jones 1983).
Consequently, more priority has been accorded to 'improving' the
character of the poor as a means of rectifying the plight of clients
than to exploring the range of social, economic and political forces
which reproduce inequalities. Historically, this orientation is exemplified in the key methods of psycho-social casework, with its focus
on remoralisation and re-education.

Even though casework is no longer the prevailing method of most
state social workers in the 1990s – the social work labour process in
state agencies has changed dramatically over the past twenty years,
with social workers being more preoccupied with gate-keeping,
rationing resources and supervision – the residual effect of that
method on social work's understanding and acknowledgment of
poverty and inequality remains. Quite bluntly, social work has operated with a blinkered outlook which downplays the significance of
the material context of poverty while maintaining an overwhelming
emphasis on the individual and on family behaviours. For all the
obfuscation that follows from this privileging of ideas, character,
morality and behaviour over the material realities of clients'
enduring poverty and their marginal relationship to the wage-labour
market, social work remains overwhelmingly a class-specific activity
concerned with some of the most evident casualties of a capitalist
society. It is so evident that, when Alvin Schorr undertook his survey
of contemporary British social work as an American outsider, he
opened his chapter on clients with the following observation:

> The most striking characteristics that clients of the personal
> social services have in common are poverty and deprivation.
> Often this is not mentioned, possibly because the social services
> are said to be based on universalistic principles. Still, everyone in
> the business knows it. One survey after another shows that
> clients are unemployed or, to observe a technical distinction, not
> employed – that is, not working and not seeking work. Perhaps

half receive income support, as many as 80 per cent have incomes at or below income support levels.

(Schorr 1992: 8)

As Schorr notes, the research evidence of clients' poverty is compelling. In the mid-1980s Becker and MacPherson (1986) discovered that nine out of ten clients were dependent on state benefits, of whom the majority were dependent on means-tested benefits. This corroborated the findings of Strathclyde's Social Work Department, which noted in 1982–3 that 90 per cent of all its referrals had social security as their main source of income (Becker, MacPherson and Falkingham 1987).

Impoverishment is a key variable in determining involvement with the personal social services. The Department of Health's Report (1991) on children coming into care noted that one in ten children aged between 5 and 9 years in families dependent on state benefits were admitted into care, compared with one in 7,000 for children in the same age group living in families not on income support. The data on all the major client groups of the personal social services, from the elderly to people with disabilities, embracing disproportionate numbers of women and Black people, reveal the centrality of poverty in the lives of those in contact with social work agencies.

The lived reality for many state social workers in the 1990s is that when they are able to free themselves from the desk-bound procedural demands of their agencies and move into the neighbourhoods of their clients, they now commonly encounter what amounts to third-world conditions. These are neighbourhoods which, Campbell noted in her 1993 study of Britain's 'dangerous places', have been abandoned by capitalism and by much of the state. They are places where even the police dare show themselves only on occasion and in force, and where people have been abandoned to survive as best they can with few publicly funded services or facilities and little in the way of legitimate paid employment. The pace of deterioration and polarisation has been dramatic. The Institute of Fiscal Studies' report (Giles et al. 1996) on shifts in social housing tenure details how in little more than a decade there has been a massive concentration of the most impoverished in the declining council-house sector; a process that might accurately be described as ghettoisation. As the Joseph Rowntree Inquiry Group on income and wealth noted, 'in many areas of the UK the living standards and life opportunities of the poorest are simply unacceptably low in a society as rich as ours' (JRF Inquiry Group, 1995).

CONDITIONAL COMPASSION

That it is possible to be disappointed by social work's response to this deepening of social inequalities and the worsening plight of those at the bottom of the social pile stems from an equally long-rooted understanding, at least among the liberal middle classes, that social work is a caring and compassionate activity that cares about the welfare of its clients. In other words, although social work organisations and professional bodies have been reluctant to acknowledge the class-specific nature of their activity, they have simultaneously proclaimed principles and commitments that indicate a concern with the plight of the poor.

However, much of the 'soft' language of social work has been confusing. Its vocabulary of care, empathy and client-centredness and self-determination, while allowing for social work's self-promotion as a caring profession, has always been ambiguous and conditional. Within the prevailing psycho-social framework of British social work, clients have been predominantly conceptualised as wayward children in need of caring control. Elizabeth Irvine, an influential British social work leader in the 1950s and 1960s, exemplified this position when she wrote that the 'great number [of clients] resemble greedy demanding children, always clamouring for material help, always complaining of unfair treatment or deprivation; this attitude shades into paranoid imagining or provoking of slights and rebuffs' (Irvine 1954: 27). Such perspectives on clients are commonplace in the social work literature, indicating a strange mixture of compassion and distrust (Jones 1997a). There is evidence of, on the one hand, concern about the problems and difficulties confronting clients and yet, on the other, of a concern that, without careful supervision, clients will unscrupulously exploit the kindness of the social worker to gain access to resources they neither deserve nor can be trusted to use to good effect. This was recently revealed by Davis and Wainwright (1996) in their research on mental health and poverty (see also Smith and Harris 1972; Rodgers 1960). They wanted to know why, despite the prevalence of poverty, mental-health workers disregarded the evident material hardships of their clients. The responses make for salutary reading and included such comments as 'if these people were given more they'd only waste it – smoking and buying luxuries rather than necessities' (Davis and Wainwright 1996: 49). They concluded that:

> Such responses firmly locate the problem of poverty and the issues it raises for daily living with individuals who use mental health services. The message is clear. Poverty is a given for service users and not a relevant issue for service professionals. The result is that service users are left not only managing the stress and strain of poverty but also the judgmental attitudes of mental health service workers. This situation is one which compounds the effects of poverty.
>
> (Davis and Wainwright 1996: 49–50)

Such conclusions reinforce John Clarke's (1993) analysis that social work's focus on individual circumstances and not on systemic and structural factors of deprivation and inequality means in general terms 'that social work has tended to reproduce rather than redress social inequality'. He continued:

> This is not to question the compassion, care and concern of individual social workers, or to suggest that individuals have not been helped by the interventions of social workers. But it is important to recognise that the position and role of social work as a social intervention was dominated by pressures to separate the alleviation of individual misery from concerns with structural inequality. This structuring of social work established constraints and limitations on the forms of help and intervention that were available to social workers.
>
> (Clarke 1993: 18)

It is little wonder, then, that social work has not generally enjoyed a positive reputation either among its clients or with the working class as a whole. In part its almost exclusive attention on the most impoverished and destitute of the working-class poor has led to social work being seen as a sign of failure; a stigmatised activity to be avoided. Moreover, once entangled with social work organisations, some clients have complained of the manner in which their lives and circumstances have been exposed to scrutiny. The handbook of the National Federation of Claimant's Unions, for example, maintained that social service departments are 'worse than the Social Security – they ask you all sorts of questions about your private life and when they refuse to pay you, there is no right of appeal' (cited Carmichael 1974: 62). Given the prevalence of these attitudes, it is understandable why so many clients come to the attention of social work agencies through third-party referrals (rather than by self-referral), and why social work is almost unique among state welfare activities in that its development and expansion has never figured in any working-class or labour movement campaign (Wardman 1977: 30).

THE PROBLEM OF SOCIAL WORKERS

Nevertheless, social work has enjoyed a reputation of being both a liberal and caring profession, if not among clients, then certainly among social workers and those who each year attempt to secure places on social-work qualifying courses. Moreover, from the mid-1970s onwards, there has been a sustained onslaught on social work from the political Right, which has identified social workers as the epitome of subversive liberal and permissive values (see Humphries 1993; Jones 1993).

The attacks on social work from the Right highlight one of the key paradoxes of social work as a state activity. While social work can be unpacked and shown to be a conservative activity, more concerned with the management of the poor than with combating poverty, social workers themselves pose a somewhat different challenge.

From the beginning of the twentieth century, core texts of British social work have addressed anxieties about the loyalty of social workers and about their acceptance of the legitimacy of social work's approach to working with the poor in a way that does not fundamentally challenge the prevailing order. The key problem of social work for the state has not been the nature of social work *per se* but rather the social workers who are expected to undertake the work. How does one ensure that – when confronted daily with the conditions and consequences of enduring poverty and suffering, on a scale which more than suggests that perhaps it is not the fault of the clients themselves – personable and largely compassionate social workers (who mainly come to the occupation out of a desire to help people) don't come to take on what are perceived as dangerously radical ideas? Or how does one ensure that, if they should develop such perspectives, they do not do anything about their contrary understandings?

However much care is taken in the selection, appointment and education of social workers to ensure that they adhere to the script of seeing poverty and suffering as a manifestation of individual or family inadequacy, such a perspective is by no means easily secured. This is made more difficult by the insistence, from the very origins of modern social work, that social workers had to be 'nice' and 'kindly' individuals.

From the COS onwards, there was an understanding that, if social work was to be effective in changing the moral outlook and behaviour of clients, this could not be achieved by punitive, aggressive or abrasive social workers. Effective social work demanded that social workers win the trust and affection of their clients and, through the ensuing relationship, persuade them by the 'personal touch', using the social worker as a role model, to bring about internal (character) change that would lead to a permanent recasting of the clients' moral outlook on the world (Jones 1978).

The personal qualities demanded of social workers, combined with the nature of their work among some of the most patently disadvantaged and impoverished, has entailed an enduring occupational history of attention to the recruitment, socialisation and regulation of social workers. The challenge of ensuring that social workers are not politically 'contaminated' by radical ideas about the reproduction of poverty and inequality as a socio-economic phenomenon has long dominated the development of British social work. Interestingly, this dimension of British social work has received very little attention, despite the fact that it could be argued to be one of the key dynamics in its development (Webb 1996). I have argued elsewhere (Jones 1978; 1983; 1989; 1996b) that the history of British social work education is in large measure a history of the regulation of social workers, driven by the concern to ensure that social workers keep to the pathologisation script and do not exploit their close contact with the casualties of society to raise fundamental questions which would challenge the legitimacy of prevailing social relations and ideology. Moreover, while social-work education has been a key site for such effort, many of the recent changes in the social work labour process, including the massive increase in proceduralism and its attendant managerialism, are driven by the same regulatory concerns.

These have not been the mere idling concerns of a few. The emergence of radical social work in the 1970s had a profound impact on the development of social work and can be identified as sharply influencing the subsequent agenda of the New Right with respect to social work policy (Jones 1996d: 12–13). The problem, as far as the Right was concerned, was not the legitimacy or value of social work as an activity which could usefully assist in the regulation and management of the most excluded and impoverished, but rather the behaviour, temperament and perspectives of social workers themselves.

It is worth noting at this point that much of the barrage of the social policy legislation which has been pushed through since 1979 has been directed at the control and regulation of state welfare professionals, rather than their replacement (see for example, Harrison and Pollitt 1994). The new regulations and procedures have impacted on the nature and character of welfare provision through, for example, limiting the autonomy and discretion of the state welfare workers. Nevertheless, the lead roles taken by teachers in education, doctors in health-care provision and so forth, while restricted by government policies, have not been replaced. This is well illustrated in the case of social work through the community care and children's legislation of the late 1980s. Neither the 1989 National Health and Community Care Act nor the 1989 Children Act seeks to squeeze out or dismantle social work. Indeed, in both of them social work, rather than being diminished is reinforced. In his analysis of the 1989 Children Act, Parton noted that:

> What is perhaps ironic in the light of all the criticisms made of social work, particularly via the child abuse inquiries, is not just that social work is still seen to have a role in the reconstructed set of balances in child protection work, but has the central role. Even though the practices and knowledge base of social work had been seen by many as untrustworthy, far from being marginalised it now, more than ever, moves centre stage. . . . it is the social services department which is the lead agency and the Local Authority social worker who is the focal professional.
>
> (Parton 1991: 212)

Similar conclusions can be drawn from the 1989 community care legislation. The fact is that social work has managed to retain a lead role within the New Right's welfare agenda, and that contrary to some concerns in the early 1980s over whether social work would survive Thatcherism, we discover that by the mid-1990s there are more social workers employed than at any other period. That is not to say that there have been no changes in state social work during the past twenty years. Rather, the argument presented here is that one of the key concerns during this epochal period of social welfare legislation and debate has been with the transformation of state social policy through the regulation of welfare workers, rather than with the dismantling of the welfare state.

CONTROLLING SOCIAL WORKERS

Although social workers were never as militant or threatening as the Right would have the public believe, state authorities and conservative commentators were shaken in the 1970s by social workers joining trade unions in unprecedented numbers, taking strike action in 1978/9, and in some celebrated incidents publicly joining with client groups to protest against the early rounds of local government expenditure cuts that followed the structural adjustment programme demanded by the IMF in 1976 (Simpkin 1979). These developments were not only unique in the history of British social work but indicated a major transformation in the character of the social work occupation: changes which suggested that social workers could no longer be viewed as entirely reliable nor left to be largely self-governing.

These developments were the result of a conjuncture of various trends and processes (Jones 1996a). The reorganisation of the personal social services following the 1968 Seebohm Report saw social work employment rapidly expand. Not only were more social worker posts created but salaries were also increased significantly, and clear career structures emerged as departments grew and managerial positions were created. Social work – which for the majority of social workers had been a vocation until that time – became a career. Whereas in the past it had been expected that, as a result of their vocation, most social workers would be prepared to work at low rates of pay (well below teachers' wages, for example) and not expect career progression, the changes which followed Seebohm reconstructed social work as a viable career option. This was particularly so for the growing number of social science graduates who were coming onto the labour market as a result of the expansion of higher education in the late 1960s. For many of these graduates, social work offered relatively well-paid and secure jobs (with prospects, especially for men) which would make use of their social science education.

The implications of these developments were felt at all levels of social work, both on the professional courses and in the agencies. Within social work education there was considerable turmoil, occasioned not only by the creation of generic social services departments but also by the challenge from within to the previously dominant casework and psycho-dynamic paradigm (see Bailey and Brake 1975). Social work was influenced by the wave of diverse critical social movements, both in Britain and further afield, between 1965 and 1975. The creation of a radical organisation, Case Con, and the increase in trade union membership and activism were both rooted in this period. It was during these years that a sustained and substantial critical literature emerged within social work itself that challenged its inattention to systemic inequalities and oppressions (Corrigan and Leonard 1981) and provided students some intellectual resources to challenge the dominant psycho-social paradigms of their courses (see Munday, 1972: 3; Jones 1978: 254–8).

Initially, the governmental agencies responsible for validating professional education took a liberal stance on these developments. In 1971 the Council for Training in Social Work (which in 1972 became part of the Central Council for Education and Training in Social Work, CCETSW) argued that it was appropriate for social-work courses to consider the structural dimensions of inequality and the purposes of the social work bureaucracies which had been created following the 1970 Local Authority Social Services Act (CTSW 1971: 19). However, within a very short time, under pressure from Local Authority employers, CCETSW significantly changed its tone. By its second annual report, it was voicing agency concern that some of the academic content of the professional courses was giving rise to the suspicion 'that the education they receive makes them difficult employees more concerned to change the "system" than to get on with the job' (CCETSW 1975: 39).

From the mid 1970s onwards, the various changes in professional social work education – from the creation of the Certificate in Social Services (CSS) to the implementation of a new professional qualification, the Diploma in Social Work (Dip SW) in 1989 – can be interpreted as marking a prevailing concern with making social workers 'safe' state employees. This has not only entailed granting employers considerable influence in the determination of the curricula (thereby reducing the influence of the colleges and universities, who previously controlled the content of social work education within the parameters laid down by CCETSW) but has also led to the imposition of a national curriculum in which the place of the social sciences has been significantly curtailed (Jones 1989, 1996b).

It is no coincidence that, at the very time when social workers were confronting more sustained inequalities and growing poverty, social work courses came under increasingly close scrutiny. Ministers were joined by agency employers in perceiving the educational components of courses, especially the social science elements, as contaminating influences (Jones 1996b). What links the accusation that social work education has been too preoccupied with the 'ologies' (sociology and psychology) and the 'isms' (racism and sexism) with the call for a curriculum based on common sense (whatever that is) is that these disciplines and issues are deemed dangerous to social workers. The danger is that it leads social workers to question critically the prevailing structures and systems of society; to suggest that some aspects of their clients' difficulties are not to be located solely within individual or family dynamics, but rather may be determined by more systemic process located in the character of contemporary British society.

What distinguishes the current period of social worker regulation is its intensity and its context. The attacks on social workers, especially in the tabloid press, have been extensive and hard-hitting (Franklin 1989), and clearly concerned with undermining the status and authority of social workers. Some of the media attacks on social workers look suspiciously as if they could have been orchestrated by Government, for example the press onslaught on the anti-racist perspectives embedded in the Dip. SW (Humphries 1993; Jones 1993). While it was permissible for the judiciary at that time to press for resources to develop anti-racism training for judges, social workers were being castigated by Government ministers and by conservative elements within social work itself for their anti-racist perspectives and initiatives. It was regarded as scandalous that social workers should be suggesting that racism was endemic in British society and that institutional racism was a significant factor in undermining the life chances and opportunities of so many Black people.

Similar outrage was apparent during the Cleveland child sexual abuse events of the late 1980s. As Campbell (1988) indicated, much of the ridiculing of the doctors and social workers involved in the case stemmed from the manner in which they drew attention to male violence against women and children, and therefore to the wider issue of patriarchal power in society. This was being done at precisely the moment when the Government was insisting that one of the key problems of run-down and impoverished council estates was the lack of fathers and the indiscipline of boys (crime) and girls (promiscuity) that ensued.

In both instances, the intensity of the onslaught and the demands for further regulation appear to have been triggered when social workers began to point to systemic features of contemporary society as being in part responsible for their clients' difficulties: in this case, racism and sexism. Needless to say, the fact that social work had for years been practised without any reference to sexism or racism attracted no official criticism, despite the overwhelming evidence that such neglect had resulted in interventions which were often hugely damaging and degrading (see Bryan *et al.* 1985: 110–120; Langan and Day 1992). But then damaging those whose lives are taken as counting for little is nothing compared to damaging the state. The former is too often tolerated, while the latter demands swift action.

Action is especially urgent at a time when the Government is intent upon shifting its relationship to the most marginalised and impoverished from practices and a rhetoric of inclusion to that of the management and regulation of exclusion (Hutton 1995). In this context, the last thing that successive Conservative governments desired were self-confident and powerful professions, such as social work, challenging the legitimacy of such a strategy at any level, or revealing its consequences for the most vulnerable and powerless in society. More specifically, with respect to social work, the reconstruction of society on market and enterprise principles demanded a fundamental shift in perspective about those who were surplus to requirements in this new set of arrangements.

THE NEW RIGHT AND SOCIAL EXCLUSION

Between 1945 and 1975 there was both a rhetoric and some actual practices within British state concerning the necessity of inclusion. Consequently, significant sections of social work's client population – especially able-bodied adults and their children – were conceived as being 'treatable', and policy was based on the view that the state, through its education, health and personal social services, should seek to ensure that they could be assisted to take their place in society as active citizens. Nurseries, community development and casework were all part of a panoply of services orchestrated to overcome the supposed deficiencies of the working-class poor and to secure their appropriate socialisation, so that they, or at least their children, could become self-sustaining and law-abiding workers.

The New Right broke sharply with this tradition of social

democracy. Free, unfettered capitalism, roaming the world without hindrance, was always going to be more brutalising to those least able to compete and survive. The social costs incurred were not to be borne by business, for fear that inward investment by transnational corporations would be lost and that those already here would transplant their operations to other locations where such costs would not be levied (Piven 1996). Moreover, it was argued, such safety-net policies not only taxed business and diminished enterprise, they demoralised the poor through weakening the work ethic and undermining social and familial responsibility.

Such a conception of the world has revitalised attitudes and perspectives which were dominant in Britain at the turn of last century. Those people pushed out of the labour market or to its margins were not only to lose services and policies that had once been concerned, in however qualified a way, with their inclusion, but they were now to be recast as a hopeless residuum. Thus a process is currently under way, both in Britain and the USA, in which some of the most impoverished and powerless of the working-class poor are no longer seen as being capable of, and requiring, rehabilitation but are being demonised as an 'underclass' (Murray *et al.* 1990; Novak 1996).

This process of reconceptualisation has important ideological and policy ramifications. Not only does it seek to legitimise the new terrain of attenuated polarisation by claiming those at the bottom of the social hierarchy are there because of moral deficiencies which place them outside the rest of humanity, it allows for the re-emergence of studied neglect. Furthermore, if intervention is required because of nuisance or social breakdown, it justifies more authoritarian and brutalising responses, with exclusion rather than inclusion as the core concern (Jones 1996c). In Britain and the USA this is probably best illustrated by the growth in the prison population and the renewed emphasis on punishment in the criminal justice systems (Raup 1996).

Against this background the lack of resistance by social-work agencies and social workers is more than disappointing and signals one of its most significant failures. As a result of the pressures – the media attacks, Government ridicule and legislative bombardment, expenditure cuts and new managerialism (Jones and Novak 1993), which in various configurations have made the job more difficult and stressful, social work appears to have abandoned its clients and capitulated in the face of the New Right's onslaught.

According to Holman (1993) the influence of the New Right has had three distinct effects on social work. 'First, it has contributed to an acceptance of poverty' (Holman 1993: 45). He contends that organisations such as the British Association of Social Workers (BASW) have largely given up campaigning around poverty and inequality, and that most social workers feel powerless in the face of poverty. Secondly, 'it has damaged the once noble concept of public service' (p. 46), and he is particularly critical of chief officers in social work agencies (in both state and voluntary sectors) who not only appear to accept 'that gross inequality is acceptable' but are prepared to take huge salaries and appear to be motivated by 'the greed of personal gain' (p. 45), rather than service to the public. Thirdly, 'social workers have offered little effective resistance to New Right intrusions into the personal social services' (p. 47).

Holman continues by citing a variety of studies which indicate that social work leaders have 'shown astonishing enthusiasm in embracing the Government's programme of minimising the Local Authority function, imposing a market culture and destroying direct provision of public services' (p. 47), and have failed to offer any resistance to the community care reforms other than make a demand for more resources. He concludes his criticisms by citing Beverly Hughes' research which 'explains that, in the face of growing poverty among elderly and disabled people, many personal social services staff have declined to expose and protest about the social deprivations and have concentrated on techniques for assessment, on managing budgets and public relations' (pp. 47–8).

ORGANISATIONAL WEAKNESS

This failure to 'expose and protest' highlights the weaknesses of professional and occupational organisation in British social work. In a current work environment which stresses obedience and compliance to the agency, in which managers are expected to manage, and where procedures are used to monitor the activity of social workers, the possibilities of protesting and exposing depend in large measure on having organisations that encourage and act upon the unique insights and experiences of social workers in ways that provide individual protection. British social work is peculiarly poorly organised when compared with other similar welfare-sector professionals, such as teachers, nurses and doctors. Since its inception in the early 1970s the British Association of Social Work has never managed to attract widespread support from social workers; although it has managed to survive, it has little in the way of presence and is a minuscule operation when compared with the Royal College of Nursing, the British Medical Association or any one of the many teachers' unions.

Although many state social workers are members of a trade union, they do not have a specialist union. Many are members of the large local government workers' union Unison (and NALGO before that), in which – although some social workers have been (and remain) active – they appear to be a minority group within the overall membership. In recent years Unison has been preoccupied with threats to local government in general, especially privatisation and cut-backs, and with the plight of the large number of low-paid employees in the sector. It has provided important protection to social workers as employees, but latterly its articulation of specific social work concerns has been spasmodic.

This lack of vibrant and organic organisation contrasts sharply with the 1970s, when social workers across the country created organisations within their unions – such as the NALGO Action Groups – or beyond – such as Case Con. The National Union of Students also organised a social work students' section, and this was active through the 1970s, running national conferences. There are now no comparable organisations.

Social work education has been similarly disappointing, and there has been a lack of leadership from this quarter. As with the world of practice, social work education has been divided between those who have more or less welcomed the New Right agenda and those who reject the intellectual gutting of the curriculum and the new roles and powers accorded to employers. Notwithstanding these divisions, social work education generally has been preoccupied with saving itself, and in so doing has been prepared to make major concessions to government in order to secure a future (at almost any cost). The retreat on anti-racism and the capitulation on the creation of a competence-based education system are but two recent examples (Jones 1993, 1996b), and a tendency among social work academics to accord the state-sponsored and funded CCETSW virtual professional status exemplifies a stupefying degree of political naiveté (Jones 1997b).

Ironically, the Government and its New Right supporters expected more resistance from such welfare professionals as social workers. Conservative intellectuals like Kristol and Moynihan (see

Steinfels 1979) were deeply concerned that such state intellectual workers, whom they classified as the 'new class', would pose an obstacle to the realisation of the New Right's agenda for transforming the state and its contract with the working class. With respect to social work in Britain, there was considerable reason for this unease, as noted above. In the event, however, neither the deepening of poverty and inequality for clients, nor measures resulting in the closer regulation of social workers, nor yet the persistent shortage of resources facing agencies have resulted in the once anticipated increase in social work resistance or opposition.

ABANDONMENT OF CLIENTS

The ultimate failure of social work has been its abandonment of its clients. State social work has survived the New Right, albeit more restricted and regulated – but the same cannot be so easily said of its clients, who are now more vulnerable and exposed than at any time since the end of the Second World War. Moreover, this abandonment does not seem to be peculiar to British social work. According to an American social work commentator:

> One would expect social workers, with the general mandate from society in serving the poor, to be at the forefront in taking on the challenge of poverty and all its manifestations. . . . It is ironic, though, that at such a time many social workers have left the public service and community arena for private and clinical practice, serving the middle classes and the 'paying public'. In the USA, where this phenomenon has been registered most strongly, and where the largest numbers of social workers is employed in the world (with over 100,000 registered members), 66% were full or part-time therapists. In 1988 . . . 86% of entering MSW students in direct service indicated their preference for private practice.
>
> (Campfens 1992: 101)

Similar trends are evident in Britain, as social workers seek employment as therapists and counsellors, or simply get out of the occupation altogether. As to the future, it is by no means clear. Social work appears capable of serving any number of masters, and, chameleon-like, can make itself useful either in the management of exclusion or in more liberal endeavours of rehabilitation. That it has such qualities should provoke serious questions. What is certain is that it cannot and should not have any role in the creation of a more socially just society until it has resolved that age old question of 'whose side are you on?'.

The absence of organisation, the loss of vision so apparent in contemporary British social work and the demoralisation of so many social workers are all features of social work's current weakness. Some of the casualties are to be found in state agencies and in the colleges and universities, but their *angst* is nothing compared with the plight of clients. In both Britain and the USA we are witnessing all the major political parties turning their backs on the excluded, claiming relative powerlessness in the face of global capitalism (Piven 1996). But this apparent powerlessness has not prevented politicians from either the Right or the Centre engaging in an escalating dialogue in which the consequences of social division and deepening inequality are met by an insistence on cutting welfare even further, as with President Clinton's chilling decision to abolish aid to families with dependent children, or further extensions to the prison system and longer sentences. Such policies, framed increasingly in the demonising vocabulary of the underclass, constitute an abandonment of the poorest and most vulnerable.

Social work is neither a revolutionary activity nor one with strong reformist credentials. However, it has long claimed a place as an element and reflection of society's humanitarian impulses. As Charlotte Towle, one of social work's internationally influential figures, once noted, 'in our social work practice we have been concerned to help people live rather than merely survive' (Towle 1956: 3). On those grounds alone, social work has a pressing responsibility to draw attention to the new and severe problems of poverty and disadvantage and to act on its:

> unique opportunity to advance the welfare of clients by calling appropriate attention to their plight with those authorities that must assume responsibility. By providing society with a more correct and overall view of the effects of poverty, social workers on the basis of observations of daily practice with their clients can turn their initially perceived powerlessness around to become an important factor for bringing about change.
>
> (Larochelle and Campfens 1992: 110)

This is a modest objective, but is it one now beyond the capacity of British social work?

REFERENCES

Bailey, R. and Brake, M. (eds) (1975) *Radical Social Work*, London: Edward Arnold.

Baldock, J. (1989) 'United Kingdom – A perpetual crisis of marginality', in B. Munday (ed.) *The Crisis in Welfare*, Hemel Hempstead: Harvester Wheatsheaf.

Balloch, S. and Hume, C. (1985) *Caring for Unemployed People*, London: Bedford Square Press.

Becker, S. and MacPherson, S. (1986) *Poor Citizens*, Nottingham, Nottingham University Benefits Research Unit.

Becker, S., MacPherson, S. and Falkingham, F. (1987) 'Some Local Authority responses to poverty', *Local Government Studies* 13(3): 35–48.

Bryan, B., Dadzie, S. and Scafe, S. (1985) *The Heart of the Race: Black Women's Lives in Britain,* London: Virago.

Campbell, B. (1988) *Unofficial Secrets*, London: Virago.

——— (1993) *Goliath: Britain's Dangerous Places*, London: Methuen.

Campfens, H. (1992) 'The new reality of poverty and social work interventions', *International Social Work* 35(2): 99–104.

Carmichael, K. (1974) 'The relationship between social work departments and the DHSS: The use of the Social Work (Scotland) Act', in M.E. Adler (ed.) *In Cash or In Kind*, Edinburgh: Social Administration Department: Edinburgh University.

CCETSW (1975) *Annual Report*, London: CCETSW.

CTSW (1971) *The Teaching of Fieldwork*, Discussion Paper No. 4, London: CTSW.

Clarke, J. (ed.) (1993) *A Crisis in Care: Challenges to Social Work*, London: Open University/Sage.

Corrigan, P. and Leonard, P. (1981) *Social Work Practice Under Capitalism*, London: Macmillan.

CRDU (1994) *UK Agenda for Children*, London: Children's Rights Development Unit.

Davis, A. and Wainwright, S. (1996) 'Poverty work and the mental health services', *Breakthrough* 1(1): 47–56.

Department of Health (1991) *Patterns and Outcomes in Child Placement*, London: HMSO.

Fox-Piven, F. (1996) 'Abdicating Power', *Red Pepper*, October: 11–13.

Franklin, B. (1989). 'Wimps and bullies: Press reporting of child abuse', in P. Carter, T. Jeffs and M. Smith (eds) *Social Work and Social Welfare Yearbook I*, Milton Keynes: Open University Press.

Giles, C., Johnson, P., McCrae, J. and Taylor, J. (1996) *Living With the State*, London: The Institute for Fiscal Studies.

Harrison, S. and Pollitt, C. (1994) *Controlling Health Professionals*, Buckingham: Open University Press.

Holman, B. (1993) *A New Deal for Social Welfare*, Oxford: Lion.

Humphries, B. (1993) 'Are you or have you ever been?', *Social Work Education* 12(3): 6–8.

Hutton, W. (1995) *The State We're In*, London: Jonathan Cape.

Irvine, E. (1954) 'Research into problem families', *British Journal of Psychiatric Social Work* 9, Spring.

Jones, C. (1978) 'An analysis of the development of social work education and social work 1869–1977', unpublished Ph.D. thesis, University of Durham.

—— (1983) *State Social Work and the Working Class*, Basingstoke, Macmillan.

—— (1989) 'The end of the road? Issues in Social Work Education', in P. Carter, T. Jeffs and M. Smith (eds) *Social Work and Social Welfare Yearbook I*, Milton Keynes: Open University Press.

—— (1993) 'Distortion and Demonisation: The right and anti-racist social work education', *Social Work Education* 12(3): 9–16.

—— (1996a) 'Anti-Intellectualism and the Peculiarities of British Social Work', in N. Parton (ed.) *Social Theory, Social Change and Social Work*, London: Routledge.

—— (1996b) 'Regulating social work: A review of the review', in S. Jackson and M. Preston Shoot (eds), *Educating Social Workers in a Changing Policy Context*, London: Whiting and Birch.

—— (1996c) 'Poverty, inequality and social division in contemporary Britain: Implications for social welfare', *Representing Children*, 9(4).

—— (1996d) 'Dangerous times for British social work education', in P. Ford and P. Hayes (eds) *Educating for Social Work: Arguments for Optimism*, Aldershot: Avebury.

—— (1997a) 'Poverty', in M. Davies (ed.) *The Blackwell Companion to Social Work*, Oxford: Blackwell.

—— (1997b) 'The case against CCETSW', forthcoming in *Issues in Social Work Education*.

Jones, C. and Novak, T. (1993) 'Social work today', *British Journal of Social Work* 23(3): 195–212.

Jordan, B. (1988) 'Poverty, social work and the state', in S. Becker and C. MacPherson, (eds) *Public Issues and Private Pain: Poverty, Social Work and Social Policy*, London: Social Services Insight Books.

JRF Inquiry Group (1995) *Income and Wealth: Report of the Joseph Rowntree Inquiry Group*, York: Joseph Rowntree Foundation.

Langan, M. and Day, L. (eds) (1992) *Women, Oppression and Social Work*, London: Routledge.

Larochelle, C. and Campfens, H. (1992) 'The structure of poverty: A challenge for the training of social workers in the North and South', *International Social Work* 35(2): 105–19.

Munday, B. (1972) 'What is happening to social work students', *Social Work Today* 3(6).

Murray, C. *et al.* (1990) *Emerging British Underclass*, Choice in Welfare Series No. 2, London: IEA Health and Welfare Unit.

NALGO (1989) *Crisis in Social Work*, London, NALGO.

Novak, T. (1996) 'The class analysis of poverty: A response to Eric Ohlin Wright', *International Journal of Health Services* 26(1): 187–95.

Oppenheim, J. (1987) 'Falling apart at the seams', *Insight*, 20 November: 10–11.

Parton, N. (1991) *Governing the Family: Child Care, Child Protection and the State*, London: Macmillan.

Parton, N. and Small, N. (1989) 'Violence, social work and the emergence of dangerousness', in M. Langan and P. Lee (eds) *Radical Social Work Today*, London: Unwin Hyman.

Raup, E. (1996) 'Politics, race and US penal strategies', *Soundings*, issue 2, Spring: 153–68.

Rodgers, B. N. (1960) 'The administration of the social services and the family caseworker' *Social Work* (USA), 17(4).

Schorr, A. (1992) *The Personal Social Services: An outsider's view*, York: Joseph Rowntree Foundation.

Simpkin, M. (1979) *Trapped Within Welfare*, London: Macmillan.

Smith, G. and Harris, R. (1972) 'Ideologies of need and the organisation of social work departments', *British Journal of Social Work* 2(1).

Steinfels, P. (1979) *The Neo-Conservatives: The Men Who Are Changing America's Politics*, New York: Touchstone Books.

Towle, C. (1956) *Some Reflections on Social Work Education*. London: Family Welfare Association.

Townsend, P. (1995) 'Persuasion and conformity: An assessment of the Borrie Report on Social Justice', *New Left Review*, no. 213: 137–50.

Wardman, G. (1977) 'Social work: A communist view', *Marxism Today*, January: 29–32.

Webb, D. (1996) 'Regulation for radicals: The state, CCETSW and the academy' in N. Parton (ed.) *Social Theory, Social Change and Social Work*, London: Routledge.

Chapter 10

Towards a classless society?

Fiona Devine

INTRODUCTION

The extent to which Britain can become a classless society, and the role of government in facilitating the emergence of a society in which class inequalities are absent, have once again entered public debate. The issue is likely be a major theme in the political discourse of the current Labour Government. Using somewhat different rhetoric, the main political parties will express their commitment to the creation of a more equal society. For the Conservative Party, these ideas will be stressed in terms of opportunities and choices. The Labour Government will emphasise new opportunities and the realisation of potential. The Liberal Democrats will call for greater opportunities and independence for all. Each party, in other words, will try to create a vision of Britain in the twenty-first century which is freed from the shackles of the class inequalities of the past. For all three parties, a classless society is defined as one in which people's life chances are achieved through merit, rather than ascribed on the basis of inherited advantage. It is a liberal view of a classless society, in which people are given equal opportunities to compete over the distribution of rewards, rather than a radical view, which also challenges inequalities of condition and outcome. It is about changing processes rather than structures (Cockburn 1991; Jewson and Mason 1986; see also Chapter 5 above).

Despite the not dissimilar rhetoric, the political parties will have different economic and social policies on which they will be judged (although some might argue that there is little to distinguish them these days). During the General Election, Labour and the Liberal Democrats were judged primarily on their visions of a better future. In contrast, as the party in office, the Conservative Party was evaluated mainly on its past record. It is a record of which the Conservative Party can hardly be proud, for it has presided over nearly two decades in which class inequalities have been heightened rather than reduced. The 1980s and 1990s have witnessed an increasing polarisation between advantaged and disadvantaged groups. There is now a large gap between the life chances of those in relatively secure employment, who have enjoyed rising standards of living, and those experiencing subemployment and unemployment, which is increasingly associated with poverty and deprivation. The growth of youth unemployment and youth homelessness is a clear manifestation of these trends (see Chapters 5 and 6 above). These trends have, in turn, generated a fear that a group of people – many of them young – are being permanently marginalised and excluded from society and reside in a dark world of crime and drugs. The growing polarisation between the advantaged and disadvantaged in society has undermined the very basis of social integration and social order. In other words, Britain is a less classless and more class-bound society than it was nearly two decades ago.

Tony Blair's new Labour Government faces an uphill task, therefore, if it is to reverse the trend towards polarisation in the 1980s and 1990s and to progress towards a classless society in the opening decade of the twenty-first century. This chapter addresses the possibilities of Britain becoming a classless society by reviewing the empirical evidence on class divisions in the second half of the twentieth century. The key questions are as follows. Did class decline in a period of economic expansion and state commitment to reducing class inequalities? What happened to class divisions in the period of economic decline and the demotion of equality as an economic and social objective? What are the implications of past patterns and trends in class inequalities for the prospect of a classless society in the future?

The rest of this chapter is divided into three sections. In the first section, the economic changes which have occurred as Britain enjoyed a period of prosperity and affluence (between 1945 and 1973) and then a period of recession and uncertainty (from 1973) are described. These, sometimes rapid, economic changes have had important implications for the social structure in British society. The middle section will draw on a wealth of empirical evidence from class analysis to examine patterns and trends in the nature of social divisions over the two periods in question. We shall see that class inequalities did not diminish in the post-war period of prosperity, and that they have sharpened in a period of economic depression and high levels of unemployment. The final section will consider the political responses to economic and social change, and the opportunities and constraints which the Labour Government will face in seeking to create a classless society. The new Labour government may be able to reverse the polarisation of class inequalities to some extent, although the possibilities of creating a more equal society are not high.

ECONOMIC RESTRUCTURING

The distribution of life chances in Britain and other industrialised societies is largely determined by the employment relations which characterise national economies. The extent to which Britain could become a classless society, therefore, can only be properly addressed by considering the changes which have occurred in the economy in the second half of the twentieth century. The period in question, 1945 to the present day, is usually split into two parts: the period of the long boom between 1945 and 1973, and the period of economic stagflation from 1973 onwards. The long boom of the post-war period was characterised by high rates of economic growth among western industrialised societies. Britain, for example, enjoyed a growth rate of 3 per cent in the 1950s and 1960s (Gamble 1994; Green 1989). It was also a period of full employment. Unemployment, in Britain, for instance, hovered below 3 per cent for much of the 1960s (Ashton 1986). National economies like Britain's grew prosperous on the basis of a huge demand in the manufacturing sector for an array of goods including cars and domestic products in an era of mass production. Of course, economic prosperity was not unchecked, for there were periods when demand fell back and unemployment grew, as in the north-east in the early 1960s. Overall, however, the period can reasonably be characterised as one of economic prosperity and affluence (Gamble 1994; Marquand 1988). This economic success generated a sense of security and optimism about the future and, indeed, led many commentators at the time to talk about the demise of class in Britain, as living standards for members of the working class rose as never before (see Devine 1992 for the debate on embourgeoisement).

The oil crisis and the Israeli–Egyptian war in the Middle East in 1973 heralded the end of the long boom. Growth rates among western industrialised countries began to slow and stutter. Britain's growth rates in the 1970s, for example, averaged between 1 and 2 per cent (Green 1989). The demand for manufacturing goods, at least in Western industrialised nations, had been met and, for example, the market for cars was saturated (Marsden *et al.* 1985). Competition became increasingly fierce across the world. As a result, unemployment started to grow steadily surpassing the (then) emotive figure of 1 million in 1972 (Ashton 1986). As the decade continued there was also growing evidence that the post-war trend towards the equalisation of wealth and income had come to an end. Indeed, the trend was reversing, so that inequality was growing (Pond 1989; Stark 1989). These trends accelerated when the deep recession of the early 1980s caused a huge shake-out of labour from manufacturing industries. Unemployment topped 3 million in 1986, while long-term unemployment rose to over 1 million (Green 1989). Unemployment was increasingly associated with poverty and deprivation, especially as state support for the unemployed was reduced so that the gap between those in employment and those out of it widened. In the late 1990s unemployment has dropped again to under 2 million, but the distribution of wealth and income remains highly unequal. For example, the proportion of people with incomes below half average income rose from 8 per cent in 1982 to 19 per cent in 1993 (*Social Trends* 1996). Again, there were times of prosperity, as with the boom of the mid-1980s, but, overall, national economies in the West have been characterised by uneven growth and increasing unemployment. Feelings of economic security and optimism have, not surprisingly, been replaced by a sense of insecurity and pessimism about the future, especially among those (predominately members of the working class) bearing the brunt of economic decline (Marshall *et al.* 1988).

It is in the context of these changing fortunes of the British economy that changing patterns of employment and unemployment need to be placed and their social implications for class inequalities subsequently understood. Commentators have identified a number of trends which have affected employment relations in the labour market. First, there has been a major change in the industrial structure of the British economy. That is, there has been a decline in the size of the manufacturing sector of the economy and a rise in the service sector. In the face of world-wide competition, technological advances and a drop in demand, manufacturing employment halved over twenty-five years. In 1966, for example, there were 8.6 million people employed in manufacturing industries, while in 1992 the

figure had dropped to 4.4 million people. The share of manufacturing employment dropped from 60 per cent in the early 1960s to
38 per cent in the early 1990s (Rowthorn 1986). The most dramatic
decline in manufacturing employment occurred in the deep recession of the early 1980s, when there were substantial losses in the
steel industry, shipbuilding, textiles and so forth. The brunt of
redundancies were born by men in semi-skilled and unskilled
manual work. In contrast, employment in the service sector – which
ranges from financial services to retail distribution – grew. The
share of service-sector employment grew from 45 per cent in the
early 1960s to 65 per cent in the 1990s. One of the major reasons for
this expansion was the growth of health and education services
associated with the emergence of the welfare state. Employment in
health and education, for example, doubled to over 3 million
between 1959 and 1981 (Allan and Massey 1988). A large proportion of these jobs have been occupied by women. The change in the
industrial sector, therefore, has been an important component of
economic restructuring.

Second, there has been a change in the occupational structure of
the British economy, with a decline in demand for manual employment and an increase in that for non-manual employment
(Gershuny 1983; Routh 1987). Occupational change has been more
gradual than industrial change, since the growth of low-level clerical work, for example, began in the early twentieth century.
However, computerisation has led to productivity gains, so that the
demand for clerical employees has dropped (Gershuny 1983).
Rather, the demand is now for high-level technical, professional and
managerial occupations. The upgrading of the occupational structure is closely associated, of course, with sectoral change. In the
context of rapid technological change, for example, there has been a
substantial demand for engineers and scientists in manufacturing
(Institute for Employment Research 1995). These occupations are
dominated by men (Evetts 1996; McRae et al. 1991). Similarly, the
growth of the service sector has been associated with increasing
demand for health and education professionals, such as doctors,
nurses, teachers and so forth. Many of these jobs are dominated by
women (Dex 1985). The growth of managers and supervisors has
been evident in both sectors. There has been a growth in low-level
service-sector employment as well, often in personal services, hotels
and catering and retail distribution. These often low-paying jobs
have been increasingly occupied by young men and women (Ashton

et al. 1990). Nevertheless, the overall trend has been towards the decline of manual employment and the growth of non-manual employment.

Third, there has been a major change in forms of employment in the face of demand for greater flexibility (Pollert 1991) There has been a decline in full-time employment, although the number of hours which full-timers work remains high, especially in comparison with other European countries (Marsh 1991). The decline in full-time employment is closely associated with the shedding of male manual workers from manufacturing. There has been a substantial increase in the numbers in part-time work. This is performed overwhelmingly by women in service-sector jobs who, in the absence of a child-care system, combine part-time employment with their responsibilities in the home. Over half (53 per cent) of women are economically active, and nearly half of them (22 per cent) work part-time (*Social Focus on Women* 1995). There has also been an increase in self-employment, which is dominated by men (also performing long hours), although the proportion of people in self-employment remains small in relation to those working as employees, whether in high-level or low-level jobs. Finally, there has been a growth in temporary or seasonal employment of various forms – although, again, this group is a small proportion of the workforce as a whole (Hakim 1988). The nature of employment, therefore, has changed considerably since the Second World War.

Finally, there is an increasing awareness of organisational change, as bureaucracies also become more flexible. The trend towards large, highly-centralised employing organisations has been reversed, as organisations have downsized into leaner operations (Clegg 1990). These changes have undermined long-standing job hierarchies and the internal labour markets of organisations. It has meant that more people – notably middle managers – now face the prospect of redundancy. There is a sense, therefore, of greater and more widespread job insecurity in the labour market as a whole (Jordan *et al.* 1992). These claims need to be substantiated over a longer time-span, and the evidence suggests that the bureaucratic career is changing but not disappearing (Halford and Savage 1995a, 1995b). In sum, therefore, full employment and job security in the 1950s and 1960s has given way to unemployment and job insecurity since the 1970s. As we shall see, however, some people have enjoyed high standards of living and a good quality of life which high-level, well-numerated employment brings, while others have experienced poverty and deprivation, which is increasingly associated with unemployment and welfare dependence. It is to the social consequences of economic restructuring – most notably the polarisation of life chances – that we now turn.

SOCIAL IMPLICATIONS

There is a substantial body of empirical research on educational and occupational mobility which has examined the extent to which class inequalities have or have not been reduced since the end of the Second World War (Goldthorpe 1980; 1987; Halsey *et al.* 1980). The results – from nationally representative survey data – are informative for they allow us to assess the possibility of Britain becoming a classless society in the foreseeable future. Goldthorpe's study of social mobility, for example, found that there has been considerable upward mobility in Britain since the late 1940s, resulting from the evolution of the occupational structure. While only 14 per cent of fathers had occupied a middle-class position, nearly twice as many sons (27 per cent) occupied the same position (Goldthorpe 1987: 59–60). The growth of the middle class also facilitated upward mobility for those of working-class origin. Goldthorpe found that over a quarter (27 per cent) of men in high-level middle-class jobs were of working-class origin. There was evidence, therefore, of substantial absolute social mobility and little evidence of closure at the top. However, when he considered relative rates of mobility, Goldthorpe (1987: 50) found 'marked inequalities in mobility chances to the disadvantage of men in working-class background'. The percentage of sons of middle-class origin reaching middle-class destinations stood at 25 per cent even though they constituted only 8 per cent of the total sample (Goldthorpe 1987: 43–5). Moreover, the sons of manual workers become 'progressively under-represented' further up the class structure, since only 16 per cent of sons of working-class origin were found in middle-class positions, compared with 60 per cent of those of middle-class origin. Thus, the sons of middle-class fathers had an almost four times better chance of getting into the middle class than the sons of working-class fathers (Goldthorpe 1987: 50). The relative chances of upward mobility, therefore, demonstrated the persistence of social closure.

Goldthorpe concluded that Britain was not an open society. Although 'more room at the top' had facilitated considerable upward mobility, it was still the case that children from advantaged social backgrounds had a better chance of advancement than children from disadvantaged homes. Moreover, Goldthorpe noted that class inequalities had remained stable despite attempts to create a more open society through educational and social policies at a time of economic expansion. These findings highlighted the limitations of the welfare state in reducing class inequalities. He concluded:

> What our results would suggest . . . is that this strategy grossly misjudges the resistance that the class structure can offer to attempt to change it; or, to speak less figuratively, the flexibility and effectiveness with which the more powerful and advantaged groupings in society can use their resources at their disposal to preserve their privileged position. There is a serious underestimation of the forces maintaining the situation in which change is sought, reactive to the measures through which, it is supposed, change can be implemented.
>
> (Goldthorpe 1987: 328)

Indeed, the failure of egalitarian reform to bring about a more equal society was hidden by economic growth in the post-war period. This conclusion was confirmed by the findings of Halsey *et al.* on the limited effect of education reform on processes of social selection. In the context of educational expansion, the absolute chances of attending university, for instance, increased while the relative chances of entry remained the same. Thus, Halsey and his colleagues concluded 'that the Education Act brought England and Wales no nearer to the ideal of a meritocratic society' (Halsey *et al.* 1980: 210; see the fuller discussion on education and class in Chapter 4 above).

Of course, there have been many criticisms of the mobility research, including those (Penn 1981; Crompton 1980) which argued that Goldthorpe and his colleagues offered an over-optimistic picture of change, and those which argued that they proffered an over-pessimistic picture of stability (Payne 1986; 1987; Saunders 1995). These debates need not concern us here. One issue of interest, however, is the extent to which the persistence of class inequalities demonstrates the failure of the welfare state. Pawson (1993), for example, has criticised Goldthorpe for his over-eagerness to leap from mobility tables to the failure of the British welfare state. It remains highly debatable, too, whether there was a clear project to reduce class inequalities with the establishment of the welfare state in 1945. The social policies of the 1945–51 Labour government were, for the most part, devised during Labour's period in the coalition government during the war. Beveridge's plans were deeply infused with liberalism and a conception of the welfare state as alleviating the worst excesses of want and squalor, rather than eliminating class inequalities as a whole (Addison 1975). It is extremely difficult to argue that post-war welfare policies have failed, for we do not know if class inequalities would have been more pronounced than they were without the welfare state. A similar argument was proposed by Blackburn and Marsh (1991) in their re-analysis of Halsey *et al.*'s data. They argued that the 1944 Education Act did have some equalising effects. They found a trend towards growing equality in the period 1944–54, but increased inequality from then on, as the baby boom population outstripped the growing number of selective places. The Act had not been entirely effective but, 'if the 1944 Act had not been in place when the baby boom generation became adolescents, class inequality would almost certainly have been very much higher than the observed level here' (Blackburn and Marsh 1991: 529–30).

Of greater interest, however, is the impact of economic recession (rather than economic expansion) on class inequalities from the mid-1970s onwards. The evidence from mobility research confirms that class inequalities have widened. Analysing mobility data from the British General Election Study of 1983, Goldthorpe found that the key findings on patterns and trends in absolute and relative rates of mobility were upheld over the period 1972–83. The opportunities for upward mobility from the working class to the middle class had continued to increase, although the middle class was also consolidating through self-recruitment – a trend confirmed by the research of Marshall *et al.* (1988) including men and women. Looking at the effects of unemployment on mobility chances, Goldthorpe found that the unemployed were predominately working-class rather than middle-class (16 per cent, compared with 4 per cent; Goldthorpe 1987: 268). The chances of upward mobility into the middle class from the working class had continued to improve since 1972, but there was also a greater risk of downward mobility for men of working-class origin as well (Goldthorpe 1987: 269). Mobility chances for men of working-class origin, therefore, had polarised with the return of unemployment. He concluded that unemployment had increased the 'stakes' in the mobility 'game' because to 'occupy a working-class position so greatly increases the risk of experiencing the rather decisive form of downward social mobility that becoming – and perhaps for long remaining – unemployed must be taken to represent' (Goldthorpe 1987: 270). Goldthorpe raised the possibility of a major social division opening up within the working class, and the 'ultimate result of such a process would be the formation of an "underclass", concentrated – and in turn isolated and fragmented – within the inner cities and the areas of most rapid industrial decay' (Goldthorpe 1987: 338). It is in this sense that class divisions polarised in the face of economic recession.

A plethora of studies in the 1980s and 1990s have confirmed that unemployment is predominately the fate of members of the working class. It was semi-skilled and unskilled manual workers who bore the brunt of job losses in the steel industry, shipbuilding and engineering in the early 1980s (see, for example, Harris *et al.* 1987; Westergaard *et al.* 1987). In localities affected by mass redundancies, like south Wales, south Yorkshire and the north-east, job opportunities have been restricted to sub-contracted work, with the prospect of further bouts of unemployment (Harris *et al.* 1987), while older men and their families have been forced into early retirement with only a future of poverty in old age (Westergaard *et al.* 1987). Young people in these areas have not fared much better, as it has proved difficult to get a foothold into the labour market (Allatt and Yeandle 1990). Youth Training Schemes, for example, have not led to jobs in depressed regions like Liverpool and Kirkcaldy as the ESRC's 16–19 Initiative showed (Banks *et al.* 1992; see also Chapter 5 above). The result has been to delay the transition from school into work and from adolescence into adulthood. Research has also indicated that unemployment – especially long-term unemployment – is associated with poverty and deprivation. The considerable financial difficulties of living on welfare payments, which have been cut back by successful Conservative governments in the 1980s and 1990s for fear of state dependence, is well-documented (Dean and Taylor-Gooby 1992; Jordan *et al.* 1992; McLaughlin *et al.* 1989). There is also growing evidence to show that unemployment is increasingly associated with poor health – lung diseases, heart problems – and ultimately early death (Wilkinson 1986). The quality of life of the unemployed, especially in the inner cities and localities in decline, is undoubtedly deprived and impoverished.

Although unemployment has now dropped below two million, the persistence of unemployment and the likely future of jobless growth has led to debate as to whether the unemployed constitute an underclass. The notion of an emerging British underclass was documented by the American sociologist Charles Murray, writing from a neo-conservative perspective in the late 1980s. Describing himself as 'a visitor from a plague area come to see whether the disease is spreading', Murray (1990: 3–4) argued, that 'Britain does have an underclass, still largely out of sight and still smaller than the one in the US. But it is growing rapidly. Over the next decade it will probably become as large proportionately as the United States' underclass. It could even become larger'. He described an underclass of working-aged healthy people distinctive in terms of their behaviour: namely, high rates of illegitimacy, rising crime and dropout from the labour market. Murray blamed the benefit system, which had bred a dependence culture, as the main cause of the underclass, and he called for a reduction in welfare as a way of reducing the growing underclass in Britain. Murray's views enjoyed the support of Conservative ministers and others – like the Labour MP Frank Field and Left-leaning journalist Melanie Phillips – who expressed their fears about an emerging underclass including young single mothers (see Page, Chapter 8) and young criminal men. In not dissimilar ways, some sociologists (Dahrendorf 1987; Halsey 1987; Pahl 1988; Saunders 1990) voiced their concern about the increasing residualisation and marginalisation of certain sections of British society. The concept of the underclass seemingly captured the feeling of the increasing polarisation of class divisions.

However, Murray's thesis in relation to the unemployed has been undermined by wide-ranging empirical evidence. Morris's (1995) local survey in Hartlepool, a town in the north-east in long-term industrial decline, certainly challenged the thesis. Examining the employment histories of a predominately working-class sample, Morris and Irwin found a variety of relationships with the labour market – long-term unemployment, temporary bouts of employment and unemployment, and relatively secure employment – not encapsulated in the concept. There was no clear division between the employed and the underemployed. That said, they found there was a tendency for skilled workers (especially those with credentials) to have chequered careers, while skilled workers without credentials and unskilled workers were prone to long-term unemployment. They concluded, 'if long-term unemployment is a feature of this class position it seems inappropriate to assign them to a separate class location, that of the underclass. To separate those affected from their position when in work is to disguise the source of their vulnerability' (Morris and Irwin 1992a: 411). Examining the social segregation of the long-term unemployed, Morris (1992) found that employment and unemployment were concentrated among family, friendship and neighbourhood networks. Given that informal means of getting a job were paramount (most notably from someone in employment), the long-term unemployed were disadvantaged in the job-search process. Thus, rather than exhibit any specific cultural predispositions towards work, it was informal patterns of association which determined success or failure in the search for employment. Similarly, Morris and Irwin (1992b) found evidence of informal exchange with kin and friends across all employment status groups, thereby undermining notions of cultural distinctiveness still further. Overall, Morris (1995: 132) concluded that the residual concept of the underclass 'runs the risk of defining unemployment as in some sense separate from class' and excludes rather than includes the unemployed in the analysis of social class.

Survey data from the Social Change and Economic Life Initiative (SCELI) indicates that the notion of the underclass – embracing a group of people who are virtually permanently excluded from the labour market – does not stand up to empirical scrutiny. That said, Gershuny and Marsh (1994: 66) found that there is 'a differential proneness to unemployment across the adult population' and 'a substantial growth in the social stratification of unemployment'. People whose parents were in low-level jobs are increasingly likely to find themselves in low-level jobs as well. A low-level job is increasingly associated with vulnerability to unemployment, especially for young men rather than young women, entering the labour market in the difficult economic climate of the 1970s and 1980s. A low occupational status explained between '30–40 per cent of all variation in months of unemployment per year' (Gershuny and Marsh 1994: 102). Gershuny and Marsh also found that an early experience of unemployment did not dominate subsequent careers, for it only explained 10 per cent of the variance in unemployment. Finally, they found that the most important influence on unemployment is the experience of unemployment in the immediate past. Unemployment, in other words, tends to be concentrated among a small group of people in low-level jobs in depressed localities. Gershuny and Marsh concluded:

There is a causal chain linking origin to occupation, and occupation to unemployment. Both links in this chain seem to be getting stronger over time. . . . [It] is quite clear that the absolute size of the gap between the unemployment experience of those in higher – and in lower-status occupations is growing: the lower in the job hierarchy, the harder-hit by unemployment. For the period 1945–85 at least, the social stratification of the experience of unemployment had been increasing.

(Gershuny and Marsh 1994: 114)

The evidence suggests, therefore, that a distinct group of people have born the brunt of unemployment and experience recurrent bouts of unemployment throughout their working lives. Moreover, the unemployed suffer from cumulative disadvantage, in that they are invariably disadvantaged in other respects, such as housing, health and family breakdown (Burchell 1994; Gershuny 1994; Lampard 1994). However, there is little evidence to suggest that this group of people are at the bottom of the pile because of their dependence on welfare. Their attitudes and behaviour do not explain why they are disadvantaged. Gallie and Vogler (1994: 126) argue that the unemployed are more committed to employment than those in work. Two-thirds (66 per cent) of employees and the self-employed would continue working even if there was no financial necessity, compared with three-quarters (77 per cent) of the unemployed. While there were variations in attitudes to work according to age (younger people being more committed than older people) and level of qualifications (the higher educated being more motivated than the less educated), the unemployed as a whole were still very committed to employment (Gallie and Vogler 1994: 130–1). Finally, there was no evidence to show that attitudes to work determined job acquisition, for those who found employment tended to be in volatile labour markets (like construction and services) with chequered careers of employment and unemployment (Gallie and Vogler 1994: 146). Overall, the evidence from the SCELI data showed that, 'we may identify a group of people with a distinct life-style at the bottom of the heap, but they were not destined to be there, and under different labour market conditions . . . they could not have been there' (Gallie and Marsh 1994: 30).

Overall, empirical research firmly shows that an adverse economic climate in the 1970s and 1980s – exacerbated by the economic and social policies of successive Conservative governments – has led to the polarisation of class inequalities in Britain. While many enjoy a good standard of living, there are others whose quality of life is poor. This conclusion is not to deny that there are important class divisions between those in work. Increasingly, income inequality and low pay also mean that there are plenty of working poor in contemporary Britain, as Westergaard (1992) reminds us. Moreover, job insecurity is a problem which is faced by those in work, although the degree of employability means that the consequences of job loss are rather different for those in high-status jobs than for those in low-status ones (Goldthorpe 1995). Nevertheless, it is not surprising that public attention has focused on the severe individual consequences of unemployment and the wider social consequences for society as a whole which follow. Thus, it is the social exclusion of the unemployed and the need to re-integrate them back into society which is deemed the most pressing political problem of the late twentieth century. It is the major issue which the political parties will have to confront if they are to reverse the trend towards the polarisation of class inequalities and to move towards a more classless society in the future.

POLITICAL FUTURES

The Conservative government had, therefore, presided over the polarisation of class inequalities in the 1980s and 1990s. Following its success at the polls in 1979 under Margaret Thatcher, it subsequently won the elections of 1983, 1987 and 1992 (the latter under the leadership of John Major (Heath et al. 1994). By the time of the May 1997 General Election the Conservative Party had been in power for eighteen years. There is plenty of evidence to suggest that the Conservative Party was not popular in office (Edgell and Duke 1991), although its success at the polls had been facilitated by a divided opposition. In 1983, as a result of internal strife – including battles with Militant – the Labour Party, under the leadership of Michael Foot, polled its lowest percentage (28 per cent) of the vote since 1918 (Heath et al. 1985; Seyd 1987; Whiteley 1983). Under Neil Kinnock the party saw a gradual improvement in its performance at subsequent elections in 1987 and 1992, but it has been a slow process – even with various policy reviews – to convince disillusioned voters to return to the fold (Heath and Jowell 1994). The internal conflict in the Labour Party in the 1980s led to the formation of the Social Democratic Party, which enjoyed popular support in the 1987 election – although this did not translate into seats, because of the first-past-the-post system. As a result of its own internal conflicts – leading eventually to its alignment with the Liberals to form the Liberal Democrats – its standing at the polls has firmly slipped. The Labour Party's high standing in the polls from the autumn of 1992 was only slightly whittled away during the General Election campaign of 1997 and it won a landslide victory, entering office on 2nd May.

The challenge for the new Government of creating a classless society is now greater than it was in the 1970s. How, then, do the political parties intend to achieve their stated objective, and will they be successful? In the 1992 Conservative Party manifesto, John Major expressed his commitment to a society in which people could be free of 'old prejudices and class barriers' and to 'encourage diversity, not division; achievement, not antagonism'. Despite the hyperbole, however, there was little in the Conservative Party's economic and social policies to indicate a strong commitment to reducing and eventually eliminating class inequalities. In the search for economic growth, the Conservative Party's primary concern was to keep inflation down, rather than reduce unemployment. Price stability is seen as the key to British industry obtaining a better competitive position in world markets. The rhetoric of supply-side economics, much favoured by Margaret Thatcher, may have gone, but the Conservative Party remains committed to the deregulation of labour markets to ensure greater flexibility – which, along with low wage-unit costs and good industrial relations, is the key to job-creation. It is only through the opportunity of the free market, therefore, that job opportunities would arise. Allied to a concern for price stability was a commitment to cutting taxes as a means of balancing the budget and controlling public spending (and thereby providing better-quality and better-value public services). Lower taxes, Conservative politicians argue, give people greater power and choice over how to spend their money. Increased opportunities, therefore, are seen in terms of rising living standards and extending personal wealth via home-ownership, share-ownership, private insurance and pensions and so on. Arguably, therefore, Conservative Party policies are designed to protect the position of the advantaged rather than improve the plight of the disadvantaged in British society. There is little substantive evidence to show that the Conservative Party is genuinely committed to Britain becoming a classless society in the future.

What was the likely fate of the unemployed under another

Conservative government? In the face of the highest recorded levels of unemployment since the 1930s, successive Conservative administrations in the 1980s devised a variety of training schemes – including the Youth Training Scheme (YTS), which gave way to Youth Training (YT) and eventually the creation of employer-led Training and Education Councils (TECs) providing young people with training according to local needs – to reduce unemployment, or (some might allege) to reduce the unemployment count (Finn 1987). The overall aim of such schemes has been to help the unemployed and long-term unemployed back into the labour market through retraining and reskilling. However, with the persistence of unemployment in the 1990s, there has been a growing preoccupation with welfare dependence (as noted in relation to debates about an emerging British underclass). This fixation has witnessed the introduction of schemes, such as Jobclubs and Job Interview Guarantee Schemes, which increasingly monitor the job-search activities of the unemployed. As part of blaming the victims for their predicament, therefore, there is now a greater surveillance of the job-search activities of the poor (Dean and Taylor-Gooby 1992). The threat of benefit withdrawal is seen as tantamount to an American-style workfare being introduced via the back door. These initiatives have been introduced against the backdrop of welfare payments – including the Social Fund to deal with emergency payments – being cut back and an increasing concern with benefit fraud. The lives of the unemployed have been further impoverished as a result. There is little evidence to suggest, therefore, that the position of the most extremely disadvantaged would be made any better under another Conservative government. On the contrary, the unemployed poor would be permanently excluded from participating in British society with wider social implications in terms of continuing polarisation and the breakdown of social cohesion.

The key question is whether the Labour Government – with its history of representing the interests of the working class – will create a classless society through an alternative range of economic and social policies. Newspaper commentary suggests there is little to distinguish the Conservative Party from the Labour Government under the leadership of Tony Blair. In some respects this claim may be true, although in other respects it is untrue. In policy documents, the Labour Party (1996) berated the way in which the Conservative Party 'has run things for the few at the top, not the many' and 'how they shrug their shoulders at the lack of social cohesion and rank injustice in the distribution of resources'. It claims, instead, to further 'the interest not of the few but of the many, the broad majority of British people'. In other words, there is no explicit mention of reducing class inequalities but a claim to create opportunities for everyone. The Labour Government is, of course, committed to economic expansion and places a strong emphasis on the new employment opportunities which will flow from sustained growth. It sets itself against *laissez-faire* economic policies. Although there is little reference to demand-led growth (the Keynesian economic policy of previous Labour governments), a more proactive role for government in modernising the economy, facilitating investment and also raising the skill and training levels of the workforce is envisaged. In these respects Labour is seeking to offer a new vision of Britain's future which is different from that of the Conservative Party. On specific policies, however, its economic policies are not altogether different from those of its Conservative opponents. The Labour Government is keen to keep inflation low, balance the budget, not raise taxes and curtail public spending. These policies did not generate economic growth under a Conservative government, and there are doubts as to whether they will lead to substantial job opportunities under the Labour Government either. Policies designed to facilitate private and public investment may improve Britain's economic performance, but it is difficult to judge how effective they would be at this juncture. Thus, Labour's commitment is to create opportunities through economic expansion, rather than carry out any fundamental redistribution through the tax and benefit system in order to create a classless society.

The Labour Government has a strong commitment to reducing unemployment – especially youth unemployment and long-term unemployment – now elected to power. Reducing youth unemployment is seen as a 'national priority' to stop the 'waste of talent and skills' as well as rising welfare bills (Labour Party 1996). It has sought to broaden the appeal of these policies by referring to the wider problem of job insecurity and the threat of job loss which pervades British society. Like the Conservative Party, it stresses the importance of education and training for the unemployed, with an additional emphasis on acquiring technological skills in the information age. Specific proposals are in place. Through a one-off windfall levy on the excess profits of the privatised utilities, the Labour Government has committed itself to getting 250,000 young people off welfare and into employment. It has proposed four options for young people: (1) jobs with a private-sector employer; (2) jobs with non-profit voluntary-sector employers; (3) full-time study; and (4) jobs on Labour's environment task force – all under the auspices of the Target 2000 scheme. Long-term unemployment will be tackled through a cash-back rebate for employers who take on those who have been unemployed for more than two years (Labour Party 1996). It will be difficult for people to remain permanently on welfare, so that a system of workfare is also envisaged under Labour. The 'problems' of the benefit trap and benefit fraud are also to be addressed. There is, therefore, a greater commitment to reducing unemployment in the Labour Government and a recognition that unemployment and poverty have wide-ranging social implications, such as crime and family dissolution. At the same time, the proposals concerning a range of education and training schemes for the unemployed are not dissimilar to those of the Conservative Party (and there are no proposals to increase benefits to the unemployed to alleviate their acute financial deprivation). Arguably, therefore, policy differences are differences of degree rather than kind. A firmer commitment to the unemployed may see some reductions in their numbers – if the demand is created – and their integration back into a 'stakeholder' society. The gap between the rich and the poor may be reduced. These policies, however, will not reduce class inequalities as a whole. Again, the creation of a classless society is a long way off.

Finally, the Liberal Democrats are not in power but they may try to influence the new Labour Government despite its huge landslide majority. Like the two main parties, they want economic growth which is sustained by long-term investment and a partnership between government and people (Liberal Democrats 1995). They want growth, of course, without inflation but with increased demand for jobs. Unlike the Conservatives and Labour, however, they are committed to raising taxes. Those who have gained under Tory rule would be asked to pay more with the introduction of a top tax rate of 50 per cent on those earning more than £100,000. It is proposed that the saving of £1.1 billion would be used to increase personal allowances and remove people at the bottom of the earnings scale. The Liberal Democrats are also committed to raising a penny on tax to boost spending on education and training. The Liberal Democrats' policies, therefore, are currently more progressive and redistributive than those of the other parties.

The Liberal Democrats, like the Labour Government, see unemployment as the 'most important social problem facing the British economy'. They also envisage reducing unemployment and bringing people back into the labour market through various education and training schemes including a voluntary 'citizens service' to exploit the talents of young people (Liberal Democrats 1995). They are committed to reforming the benefits system to meet this end. The Party advocates the introduction of a Benefit Transfer Scheme which would mean that social-security benefits payable to the long-term unemployed could be converted to vouchers payable to employers who took them on. The maximum initial value of the voucher would be £150 per week reducing by £150 for each week of employment, thereby avoiding an open-ended commitment (Liberal Democrats 1994). The extent to which employers would see benefits in the scheme and provide new opportunities for employment remains open to debate. Whether the repackaging of benefits in this manner, therefore, would get the unemployed back to work and reduce the polarisation of class divisions in British society remains to be seen, but, without electoral success, these policies are unlikely to be put into practice.

Overall, the prospects for a classless society – in which today's young people can enjoy equal life chances in education, work, housing, health and so on – do not look good. The Labour Party, now in power again after 18 years, is committed to reversing the trend towards the polarisation of class inequalities which characterised the 1970s and 1980s. It may be able to reverse this trend by reducing unemployment and the poverty now so closely associated with unemployment, although, in an ever-competitive global economy, it will not be easy to do so. The Labour Government will probably not be able to eliminate unemployment altogether, so there is the challenge of providing support for the unemployed, so that they too can enjoy a decent standard of living. This issue has yet to be seriously addressed. Finally, in the context of growing inequality in the distribution of wealth and income, the challenge of improving the position of the working poor through the tax system, the minimum wage, employment protection and so forth, has yet to be tackled head on. In other words, the Labour Government has a restricted view of the welfare state acting as a safety-net for the unfortunate but it does not have an expansive vision of how the tax and benefit system could be used to redistribute wealth and income more equally in British society. The trend towards the polarisation of class divisions may be reversed, therefore. If so, Britain could return to the level of inequality which existed before the 1980s, thus becoming a more equal society than it is today, but the prospects for creating a classless society in the twenty-first century are slim.

CONCLUSION

In this concluding chapter, the question of whether Britain could become a classless society – and the role of government in facilitating a classless society – has been addressed. Along with the other chapters in this book, this issue has been considered with specific reference to young people and the extent to which they will enjoy equal life chances in all aspects of their daily lives. We saw that the onset of an adverse economic climate in the early 1970s and the, sometimes rapid, restructuring of the economy has witnessed the re-emergence of high levels of unemployment in particular and widespread job insecurity in general. These economic changes have had far-reaching social implications, polarising class divisions between the advantaged and the disadvantaged who now have a very different quality of life. The starkest example, which is not difficult to imagine, is that of a young person (often from an advantaged background) who enjoys the benefits of the education system before entering a well-remunerated professional or managerial occupation as opposed to the young person (often from a disadvantaged background) who gets little from the education system and faces the prospect of low-paid employment and bouts of unemployment. The outlook for young people's lives, therefore, can be very different. These socio-economic trends have been exacerbated by successive Conservative administrations which have cut public spending on welfare to the extent that unemployment is increasingly associated with poverty and deprivation. The depth of this poverty has led to widespread concern about the problems of social exclusion and the need to reintegrate the unemployed back into society. There is an increasing realisation that unemployment does not only have individual consequences but wider social consequences for the whole of society as well. The polarisation of class divisions and the evidence of poverty amidst affluence is a sign that Britain has become a more impoverished society over the last twenty years.

The Labour Government, committed to a classless society, is, therefore, faced with the huge task of, firstly, reversing the trend towards polarisation and, secondly, creating a more equal society overall. John Major may have expressed his desire for the Conservative Party to create a more classless society but its economic and social policies have worsened class divisions rather than eliminated them. There is little evidence, from the Conservative Party's record in office, that its commitment to a classless society is anything more than rhetoric. Given its history as the party which represents the interests of the working class, the Labour Party is more committed to a classless society than the Conservative Party. That said, it seeks to achieve equal opportunities through economic expansion and an increased demand for jobs which would help the unemployed back into work. The Labour Government may achieve its objectives although there are serious doubts as to whether Britain can achieve the economic growth and full-employment which characterised the long boom. Moreover, economic expansion does not guarantee greater equality. The creation of jobs in the United States under President Clinton, for example, has been accompanied by growing income inequality and increased poverty rates. Given its concern to contain public expenditure, the Labour Government has been silent on how the tax and benefit system might be used as a redistributive lever for greater equality. The Liberal Democrats are more forthcoming in this respect – although, arguably, their radicalism derives from the knowledge that they are unlikely to obtain political power. Likely government actions to facilitate a classless society, therefore, appear to be rather modest. The prospect of a classless society in which today's young people might enjoy equal life chances is in the distant rather than the immediate future.

REFERENCES

Addison, P. (1975) *The Road to 1945*, London: Jonathan Cape.

Allan, J. and Massey, D. (eds) (1988) *The Economy in Question*, London: Sage.

Allatt, P. and Yeandle, S. (1990) *Youth Unemployment and the Family*, London: Routledge.

Ashton, D. (1986) *Unemployment under Capitalism*, Brighton: Harvester.

Ashton, D., Maguire, M. and Spilsbury, M. (1990) *Restructuring the Labour Market*, London: Macmillan.

Banks, M., Bates, I., Bracewell, G., Bynner, J., Emler, W., Jamieson, L. and Roberts, K. (1992) *Careers and Identities*, Buckingham: Open University Press.

Blackburn, R.M. and Marsh, C. (1991) 'Education and social class:

Revisiting the 1944 Education Act with fixed marginals', *British Journal of Sociology*, 42: 507–36

Burchell, B. (1994) 'The effects of labour market position, job insecurity and unemployment on psychological health', in D. Gallie, C. March and C. Vogler (eds) *Social Change and the Experience of Unemployment*, Oxford: Oxford University Press.

Clegg, S. (1990) *Modern Organisations*, London: Sage.

Cockburn, C. (1991) *In the Way of Women*, London: Macmillan.

Conservative Party (1992) *The Best Future for Britain*, London: Conservative Party.

Crompton, R. (1980) 'Class mobility in modern Britain', *Sociology*, 12: 117–19.

Dahrendorf, R. (1987) 'The erosion of citizenship and its consequences for all us', in *New Statesman*, 12 June, 12–15.

Dean, H. and Taylor-Gooby, P. (1992) *Dependency Culture*, Hemel Hempstead: Harvester Wheatsheaf.

Devine, F. (1992) *Affluent Workers Revisited*, Edinburgh: Edinburgh University Press.

Dex, S. (1985) *The Sexual Division of Labour*, Brighton: Wheatsheaf.

Edgell, S. and Duke, V. (1991) *A Measure of Thatcherism*, London: HarperCollins.

Evetts, J. (1996) *Gender and Career in Science and Engineering*, London: Taylor and Francis.

Finn, D. (1987) *Training Without Jobs*, London: Macmillan.

Gallie, D. and Marsh, C. (1994) 'The experience of unemployment', in D. Gallie, C. Marsh and C. Vogler (eds) *Social Change and the Experience of Unemployment*, Oxford: Oxford University Press.

Gallie, D. and Vogler, C. (1994) 'Unemployment and attitudes to work', in D. Gallie, C. Marsh and C. Vogler (eds) *Social Change and the Experience of Unemployment*, Oxford: Oxford University Press.

Gamble, A. (1994) *Britain in Decline*, 4th ed., London: Macmillan.

Gershuny, J. (1983) *Social Innovation and the Division of Labour*, Oxford: Oxford University Press.

—— (1994) 'The psychological consequences of unemployment: an assessment of the Jahoda thesis', in D. Gallie, C. Marsh and C. Vogler (eds) *Social Change and the Experience of Unemployment*, Oxford: Oxford University Press.

Gershuny, J. and Marsh, C. (1994) 'Unemployment in work histories', in D. Gallie, C. Marsh and C. Vogler (eds) *Social Change and the Experience of Unemployment*, Oxford: Oxford University Press.

Goldthorpe, J.H. (1995) 'The service class revisited', in T. Butler and M. Savage (eds) *Social Change and the Middle Classes*, London: UCL Press.

—— (in association with C. Llewellyn and C. Payne) (1980) *Social Mobility and Class Structure in Modern Britain*, Oxford: Clarendon Press.

—— (in association with C. Llewellyn and C. Payne) (1987) *Social Mobility and Class Structure in Modern Britain*, 2nd ed., Oxford: Clarendon Press.

Green, F. (ed.) (1989) *The Restructuring of the UK Economy*, Hemel Hempstead: Harvester Wheatsheaf.

Hakim, C. (1988) 'Trends in the flexible workforce', in *Employment Gazette*, 95: 549–60.

Halford, S. and Savage, M. (1995a) 'Restructuring organisations, changing people: Gender and careers in banking and local government', *Work, Employment and Society*, 9: 97–122.

—— (1995b) 'The bureaucratic career: Demise or adaption', in T. Butler and M. Savage (eds) *Social Change and the Middle Classes*, London: UCL Press.

Halsey, A.H. (1987) 'Social trends since World War II', in *Social Trends* 17: 11–19.

Halsey, A.H., Heath, A. and Ridge, J. (1980) *Origins and Destinations*, Oxford: Clarendon Press.

Harris, C.C. and the Redundancy and Unemployment Research Group (1987) *Redundancy and Recession in South Wales*, Oxford: Basil Blackwell.

Heath, A. and Jowell, R. (1994) 'Labour's policy review', in A. Heath, R. Jowell and J. Curtice, with B. Taylor (eds) *Labour's Last Chance?*, Aldershot: Gower.

Heath, A., Jowell, R, and Curtice, J., with Taylor, B. (eds) (1994) *Labour's Last Chance?* Aldershot: Gower.

Heath, A., Jowell, R. and Curtice, J., with the assistance of J. Field and C. Levine (1985) *How Britain Votes*, Oxford: Pergamon.

Institute for Employment Research (1995) *Review of the Economy and Employment*, Coventry: University of Warwick.

Jewson, N. and Mason, D. (1986) 'The theory and practice of equal opportunities policies: Liberal and radical approaches', *Sociological Review*, 34: 229–51.

Jordan, B., James, S., Kay, H. and Redley, M. (1992) *Trapped in Poverty?*, London: Routledge.

Labour Party (1996) *New Labour, New Life for Britain*, London: Labour Party

Lampard, R. (1994) 'An examination of the relationship between marital dissolution and unemployment' in D. Gallie, C. Marsh and C. Vogler (eds) *Social Change and the Experience of Unemployment*, Oxford: Oxford University Press.

Liberal Democrats (1994) *Working for Change*, Policy Paper 9, London: Liberal Democrats.

Liberal Democrats (1995) *Investment, Partnership, Sustainability*, Policy Paper 16, London: Liberal Democrats.

McRae, S., Devine, F. and Lakey, J. (1991) *Women into Engineering and Science*, London: Policy Studies Institute.

McLaughlin, E., Millar, J. and Cooke, K. (1989) *Work and Welfare Benefits*, Aldershot: Avebury.

Marquand, D. (1988) *The Unprincipled Society* (1988) London: Jonathan Cape.

Marsden, D., Morris, T., Willman, P. and Wood, S. (1985) *The Car Industry*, London: Tavistock Publications.

Marsh, C. (1991) *Hours of Work of Women and Men in Britain*, London: EOC/HMSO.

Marshall, G., Rose, D., Newby, H. and Vogler, C. (1988) *Social Class in Modern Britain*, London: Unwin Hyman.

Morris, L. (1992) 'The social segregation of the long-term unemployed in Hartlepool', *Sociological Review*, 38: 344–69.

—— (1995) *Social Divisions*, London: UCL Press.

Morris, L. and Irwin, S. (1992a) 'Employment histories and the concept of the underclass', in *Sociology*, 26: 401–20.

—— (1992b) 'Employment and informal support: Dependency, exclusion or participation', in *Work, Employment and Society*, 6: 185–207.

Murray, C. (1990) *The Emerging British Underclass*, London: Institute of Economic Affairs.

Pahl, R. (1988) 'Some remarks on informal work, social polarisation and the social structure', in *International Journal of Urban and Regional Research*, 12: 247–67.

Payne, G. (1986) *Mobility and Change in Modern Britain*, London: Macmillan.

—— (1987) *Employment and Opportunity*, London: Macmillan.

Pawson, R. (1993) 'Social mobility', in D. Morgan and L. Stanley (eds) *Debates in Sociology*, Manchester: Manchester University Press.

Penn, R. (1981) 'The Nuffield class categorisation', in *Sociology*, 15: 265–71.

Pollert, A. (ed.) (1991) *Farewell to Flexibility?*, Oxford: Basil Blackwell.

Pond, C. (1989) 'The changing distribution of income, wealth and poverty', in C. Hamnett, L. McDowell and P. Sarre (eds) *The Changing Social Structure*, London: Sage.

Routh, G. (1987) *Occupations of the People of Great Britain, 1801–1981*, London: Macmillan.

Rowthorn, B. (1986) 'Deindustrialisation in Britain', in R. Martin and B. Rowthorn (eds) *The Geography of Deindustrialisation*, London: Macmillan.

Saunders, P. (1990) *Social Class and Stratification*, London: Routledge.

—— (1995) 'Might Britain be a meritocracy?', in *Sociology*, 29: 23–41.

Seyd, P. (1987) *The Rise and Fall of the Labour Left*, London: Macmillan.

Social Focus on Women, (1995) London: CSO/HMSO.

Social Trends 26 (1996) London: CSO/HMSO.

Stark, T. (1989) 'The changing distribution of income under Mrs Thatcher', in F. Green (ed.) *The Restructuring of the UK Economy*, Hemel Hempstead: Harvester Wheatsheaf.

Westergaard, J. (1992) 'About and beyond the underclass: Some notes on influences on social climate on British sociology today', in *Sociology*, 26: 575–867.

Westergaard, J., Walker, A. and Noble, I. (1987) *After Redundancy*, Cambridge: Polity Press.

Whiteley, P. (1983) *The Labour Party in Crisis*, London: Methuen.

Wilkinson, R. (ed.) (1986) *Class and Health*, London: Tavistock.

Index

86–7; Germany 78; government
resources 124; government
schemes 90; industry funds 79;
national scheme 76; National
Traineeships 92; skills 82; young
single mothers 168–9; youth 18,
72–95, 98–9; *see also* youth
training
Training Agency 86
Training Commission 86
Training and Education Councils
(TECs) 216
Training and Enterprise Councils
(TECs) 88–9; Youth Credits 92
'try-out schemes', youth 81

under-achievement, material
deprivation 59
underclass 4, 5, 27–31; attitudes 28;
behaviour 27; Black youth 30;
Clarke's statement 29; definition
6; EU 86; social exclusion 146;
unemployment 212; USA 193,
211; working class 193
underemployed 211
unemployment: 1980s/1990s studies
210; choice 23; economy 204;
education 86; graduates 100;
reduction 217; underclass 212;
working-class families 109;
young people 18–21, 56; youth
98, 99, 202; YTS 80–1
Unison union 195
United States of America (USA):
job creation 221; social division
197; social work 196; street
children 112; underclass 193,
211; young single mothers 173;
youth crime 144
universities, gender differentials 64
Unmarried Mother and her Child,
National Council for the
153, 157
unmarried mothers *see* lone
parents; mothers; single
mothers; women

violence, increase 28

vocabulary: care 184; *see also*
language
vocations: course titles 84;
qualifications 75, 90–1
voucher system, nursery education
52, 53
vulnerability: Housing Acts 110,
111; single homeless persons
103; working-class 179

wages: 1970s trend 19; expectation
23; golden key 108; low 19;
minimum 9
Wages Council: abolition 99; young
people 19
Wainwright, S. 184–5
'warehousing sector', young people
82, 83
wealth: children 14; equalisation
204; redistribution 122
Weber, M. 4, 5
welfare: benefits 105–9, 163;
dependence 151; French
comparison 136; Labour Party
217; New Right 188; single
mothers 155–7, 159, 163; social
work 186; spending cuts 220
West, P. 16
Westminster Council, nursery
education 51–2
Williamson, H. 30–1, 33
women: service sector 206; under 20
births 160, 161; *see also* Child
Support Act; mothers; single
mothers; prostitution
work: discipline 23; redistribution
122; standards in Britain 87
workfare scheme 171–2, 216, 218
working class 1; academia 69;
collectivism 67; education 17, 59;
employment histories 211; full-
time education 66; government
policy 33; inequalities 20;
mothers 154, 155;
neighbourhoods 121; social
work 185; socialisation 192;
underclass 193; unemployment